THE BACK PAIN BOOK

A Video Assisted Back Pain Relief Book with Back
Pain Exercises for Those Over 50

CHRIS RAWSON

Contents

Introduction

I have a vivid memory from when I was only 15 years old, of my father approaching the sidelines of my football (soccer) match after his doctor's appointment for his chronic back pain. He was using a stick that doubled up as a seat as he wasn't able to stand for any period of time. It really threw me seeing my dad who was merely in his mid-40's already having to use a mobility aid. I felt helpless that he was in that state and there was nothing I could do about it. At the time, of course, I can't say I knew that this was exactly what sparked my interest in physio, but I do remember how it made me feel. I wanted to help him, and I wanted to heal his pain.

Fast forward a few years, and I'm in the middle of my A-levels, trying to decide what subject to study at university. I have always been passionate about sports, exercise, and health, and at the same time, knew I wanted to help people in the same way I had wanted to help my father a few years prior. While wandering around a career fair at school, I stumbled upon the physiotherapy stall where a few current and graduated students were speaking. I got to understanding what physios do on a day-to-day basis, and it got me thinking that it might actually be the way that I can help people directly. Not only would it allow me to utilize my passion for exercise and health, but it would also allow me to help people improve their pain, like I wanted to help my father. From that moment on, I knew I wanted to be a physio.

Although I was only 18 at the time, my interest in helping and healing transformed into much more than I ever thought possible throughout my time at university. The human body is fascinating, and it was exciting to be fully immersed into a world of anatomy and physiology, both educationally and clinically. I couldn't wait to graduate and start my official work, and to finally help my father with his ongoing chronic pain. I have since worked for 6 years as a qualified physiotherapist in London, both within the National Health Service (NHS) in the UK, and also privately through my own business. To my surprise, the more patients I saw, the more I realized that my father was simply one of millions of people in the UK suffering from some form of back pain.

Back pain has essentially grown to be an epidemic problem in the Western world, and this is odd considering we are in a time when our medical care has never been more advanced. Our bodies are adjusting to a much more sedentary lifestyle than that of our ancestors who were steadily active, searching for food and running from predators. Our bodies evolved to move. We now live a modern lifestyle that our ancient bodies were not meant to– sitting at desks for prolonged periods of time, or performing repetitive motions in career fields that put wear and tear on our backs. Back pain has become a leading cause of disability in Western societies, and it often prevents people from performing simple daily tasks or even going to work.

However, from my personal patient experience, many cases of back pain can be highly diminished and even cured, through consistent application of holistic rehabilitation programs. The general causes of chronic back pain are often misconceived by both the medical field, and those who are suffering. While it is true that pain is often caused *initially* by some sort of injury, the pain *persists*, due to the tightening of muscles and the imbalances this causes in the body. Pain can also have certain triggers, like bending, lifting, or even sneezing, and when you determine your own triggers, you can learn to avoid them and manage them. Of course, certain conditions are more complicated and are not necessarily caused by certain triggers alone, but it's still possible to improve pain using a holistic approach.

When muscle imbalances exist in the body, unnecessary tension is placed on muscles in the back, constantly pulling on the spine in one direction or the other. Not only can this cause muscular pain and discomfort, but it can also compress nerves and cause other spinal abnormalities. On top of this, stress– about the pain itself, disappointment about lack of improvement, and/or other life anxieties–is added into the mix which only makes the muscle tension and pain even worse (more about this later).

Many treatments try to cure or dull the pain itself through prescription medications, injections, or advising the patient to simply rest and hope it eventually goes away. Yet, these things never seem to work, and it's only a matter of time before patients find themselves back in the clinic with the same or worse pain because the root cause of the pain is often overlooked–the pain is merely a symptom of the actual problem.

I know that when you've been living in pain for a certain amount of time, it can be nearly impossible to remember what it feels like to live without it. With this book I'll show you some possible causes for your back pain, and I'll provide you with the knowledge and customizable programs that will allow you to manage your symptoms. Through the 7-step holistic approach that I present in this book, I believe anyone can put themselves in the best possible position to manage their pain. Immerse yourself in this book and soak up all the information it has to offer. I hope that *Back to Basics* will empower you to start–and stick with–your journey of managing your pain.

All the best,

Chris Rawson, Physiotherapist, BsC Hons

Why Over 50's:

In my time as a physiotherapist, the age group that I have always gravitated towards for treating was those over the age of 50. This might be a sweeping statement (luckily those under 50 probably won't be reading this), but over-50's tend to be much better listeners, taking in as much information as possible to better themselves. They are inquisitive and ask (sometimes challenging) questions and by and large are the most diligent people when it comes to actively performing their exercises. From my time working in the NHS and in private practice, it appeared all too often that this age demographic was told in no uncertain terms, that "there's nothing that can be done for you–it's just wear and tear." Sound familiar?

When I was 24 years old, I decided to embark on a challenge and set up my own mobile physiotherapy service, specializing in treating just those over the age of 50. Two years later, I thought I'd take on the even greater challenge of putting pen to paper and putting everything I have learned into a book–this book. There are several books out there which cover managing back pain in great detail, however there are none, to the best of my knowledge which specifically aim to help those over the age of 50 understand their back and more importantly manage their back pain. So without further ado, read on, absorb the info, and hopefully, by the end of this book, you will have the tools necessary to improve your back pain, and improve your quality of life.

How to Use This Book For Your back

Since graduating with my physiotherapy degree my desire has been to design a more *efficient* way for treating back pain, and one that could be applied to the majority of back conditions (I say majority, as there are some that will need medical intervention, which I will explain in the next chapter). I have learned that there are 7 key areas you need to address if you want to have the best shot at successfully treating or managing your back pain. Although all back conditions vary in terms of their symptoms, all have the same basic requirements to improve their associated symptoms.

The first two chapters will help you as the patient to gain a better understanding of your back and the treatment options available to you, should you need them. Chapter 3 focuses on how important posture is for your back pain and some really useful easily applicable tips you can implement straight away to help. Chapters 4, 5 and 6 are really key, as the focus of these chapters are the stretching, strengthening, and cardiovascular components that you can include in your program. If there are exercises that are not recommended for your condition, then it will be clearly stated. However, for whatever type of back pain you have, all 3 components (stretching, strengthening, and cardio) are completely essential to managing your pain, and should be implemented regularly. The final chapter looks beyond exercise, and presents other areas that could be heightening your pain and explains how to address these. In addition to the exercise programs, the information in the last chapter can have a big impact on your mental state, allowing you greater control over your pain.

The exercise plan is as follows. Keep it in mind as you are reading so that you can determine which stretches and exercises you'd like to implement for each day.

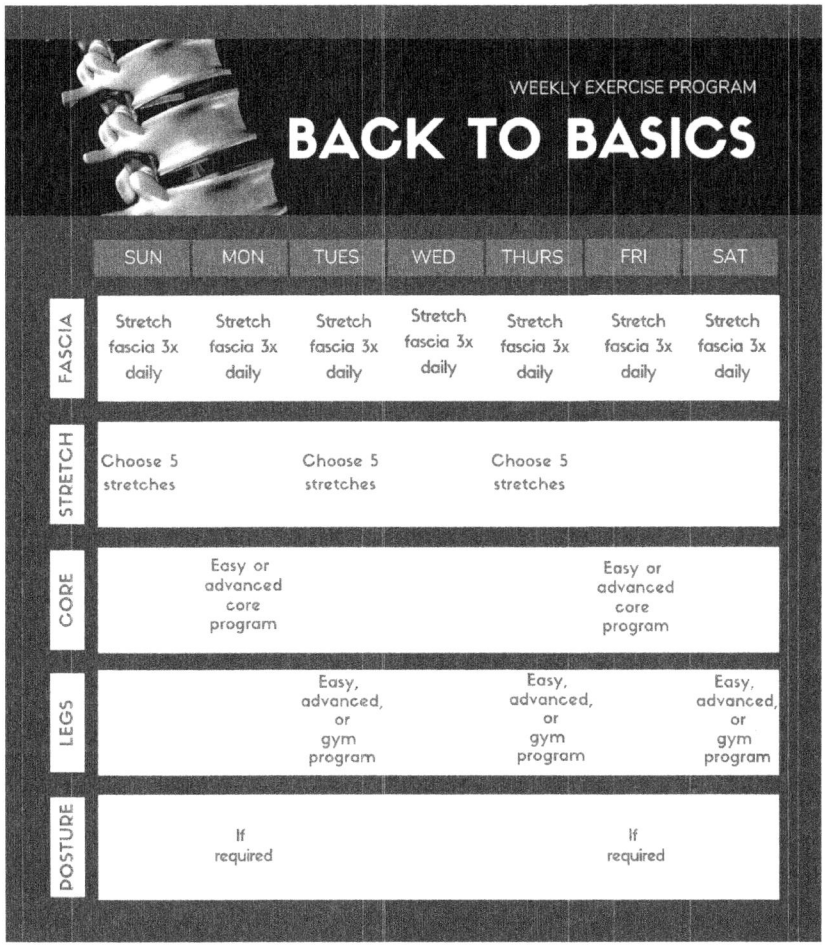

WEEKLY EXERCISE PROGRAM
BACK TO BASICS

	SUN	MON	TUES	WED	THURS	FRI	SAT
FASCIA	Stretch fascia 3x daily	Stretch fascia 3x daily	Stretch fascia 3x daily	Stretch fascia 3x daily	Stretch fascia 3x daily	Stretch fascia 3x daily	Stretch fascia 3x daily
STRETCH	Choose 5 stretches		Choose 5 stretches		Choose 5 stretches		
CORE		Easy or advanced core program				Easy or advanced core program	
LEGS			Easy, advanced, or gym program		Easy, advanced, or gym program		Easy, advanced, or gym program
POSTURE		If required				If required	

Don't forget–I have created supplementary videos to go alongside the book. These were made to help you learn proper form and help you feel confident when performing the exercises and stretches. I hope you will utilize them!

To access them, simply click on the following link or head over to:

basics.chrisrawsonphysio.com

Step 1: Get to Know Your Back

I HAVE FOUND that having a good understanding of the basic anatomy of the back and the different muscles you are trying to strengthen or stretch can be an extremely important measure in how someone manages their back pain. This is something I never thought I would have preached when I finished my university degree, as I thought it was my sole responsibility to give patients what I thought they needed and whether they knew why they were doing an exercise or not didn't make a difference. It was only when I really started to ensure my patients knew exactly *why* they were doing a certain exercise, and that they were more aware of the basic anatomy of the back, that they showed overall improvement in managing their back pain.

ANATOMY OF YOUR BACK

When I first started to treat people suffering with back pain, I was always confused by the lack of knowledge people had about their back and the anatomy of the spine. Then of course I realized that anyone who's not a physio, a doctor, or some other form of medical professional, wouldn't need to know about the muscles and joints of the back or the different types of posture. I only know the ins and outs of anatomy because it's my job, and I've spent years learning as much as I possibly could, and will continue to do so as long as I'm in practice. As I said, I've found that those with at least a basic understanding of how the back works were at a much better starting point in managing their back pain. This is by no means a call for you to invest in all the anatomy books known to man, but a well-rounded, fundamental understanding goes a long way. Let's cover the basics!

Spinal Column: Also known as your backbone or vertebral column, your spinal column is made up of a collection of 33 vertebrae, and its role is to provide structural support for your whole body. It is also essential at providing protection for the spinal cord which travels through the hollow parts of each vertebrae.

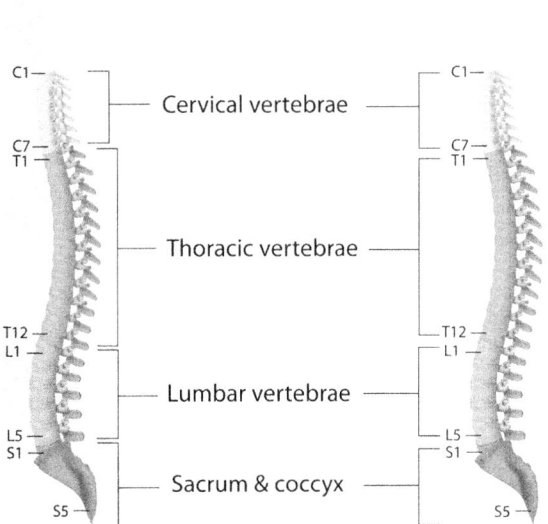

| The Vertebral Column

Vertebrae: A vertebra is the name given to each singular bone in your spinal column (vertebrae is plural for all of the vertebra). There are 24 articulating bones in the vertebral column. 7 are in the neck (**cervical spine**), 12 are in the upper and middle parta of your back (**thoracic spine**) and 5 make up your lower back (**lumbar spine**).

*You may have heard medical professionals use the terms L1 or T12 or C6, this all relates to the vertebrae number on the spine as pictured above.

Cervical Spine: The section of vertebrae that make up your neck. These are the smallest, but allow for a large range of motion.

Thoracic Spine: This is the section of the spine that makes up the mid-to-upper portion of the back, starting at the base of the neck (cervical spine). The vertebrae here are larger than the cervical. Each vertebra has two ribs attached to it on its right and left side.

Lumbar Spine: This is the lowest section of the spine, sitting in the lower back. The lumbar spine vertebrae are the largest of all, as they have to withstand the most force and pressure.

Sacrum: The sacrum is end of your spinal column and sits just below the lumbar spine. It is made up of 5 fused bones.

Coccyx: This sits just below the sacrum, and again, is made up of fused bones, this time between 2-4 vertebrae are fused together.

Intervertebral Discs: Between each of the vertebral bodies lies what are called intervertebral discs ("inter" simply means in-between). These discs are spongy circular pads and are made up of two parts. There is the **annulus fibrosus** which is an outer layer of collagenous ring giving the disc it's tough exterior and maintaining its circular shape. The inside of the disc is what is known as the **nucleus pulposus,** which is the inner, squidgy part of the disc, and it is full of nutrients. The intervertebral discs have two main roles: they allow for a large amount of movement of the spinal column, and they act as shock absorbers for the spine by distributing a large volume of load evenly through the column. They are very prone to injury, which we will go through in Chapter 2.

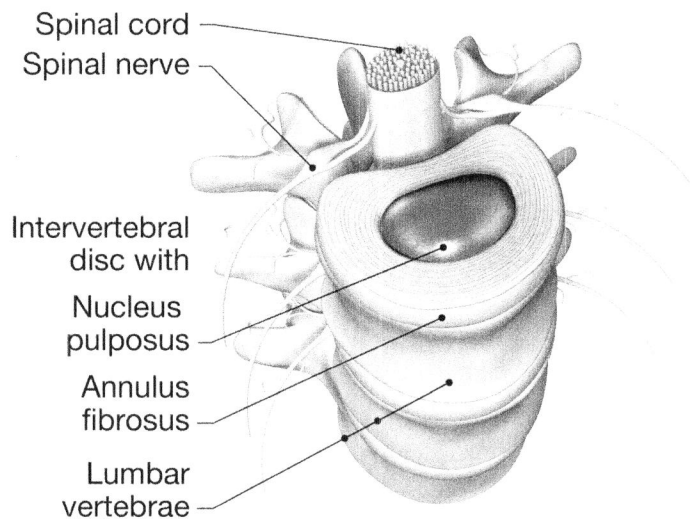

Spinal cord
Spinal nerve

Intervertebral
disc with

Nucleus
pulposus

Annulus
fibrosus

Lumbar
vertebrae

Intervertebral discs, showing annulus fibrosus and nucleus pulposus

Facet Joints: These small joints of the back run up the side of the whole spine, with one on either side of the vertebral body. They allow for rotation of the spine and are a common site of injury in your back.

Pelvis: While this technically doesn't form part of your spine, it is very commonly involved with lower back issues. It is made up of your sacrum and your hip bones, forming the pelvic girdle.

Sacroiliac Joint: This is a very commonly injured joint. There is a right and left sacroiliac joint and it is simply where your sacrum joins with your pelvic bones.

The Pelvic Girdle

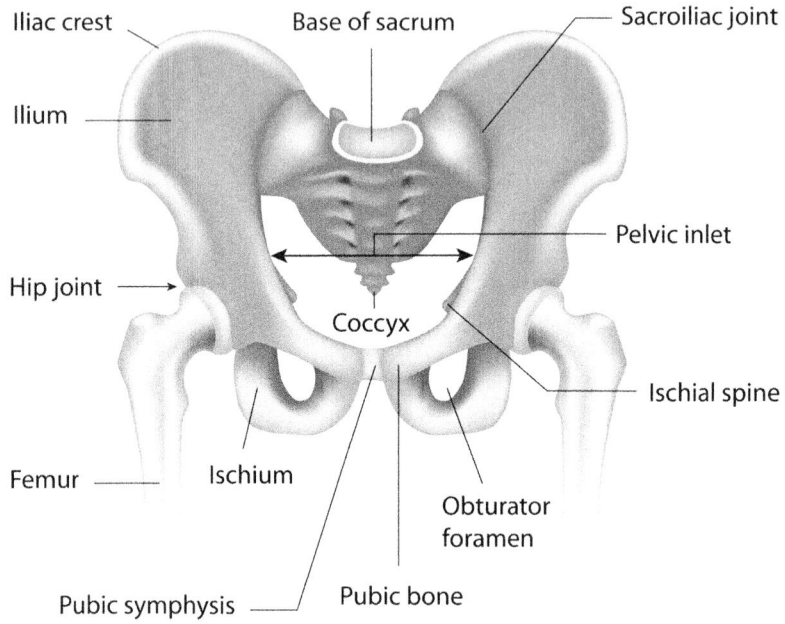

Iliac crest · Base of sacrum · Sacroiliac joint · Ilium · Pelvic inlet · Hip joint · Coccyx · Ischial spine · Femur · Ischium · Obturator foramen · Pubic symphysis · Pubic bone

Nerves: The spinal cord runs up the back part of the spinal column through a hollow opening in each of the vertebra, called the vertebral foramen. At each 'level' (each vertebra), the spinal cord branches off with individual nerves that supply various parts of the body, and these are called **nerve roots**. The lumbar spine nerves exit the lumbar spine levels and supply your lower extremities. The thoracic spine nerves supply the midsection of your body and finally your cervical spine nerves supply your upper body.

Sciatic Nerve: The nerve roots (L4-S3) of the lower back converge together to form the sciatic nerve. This starts from the back and runs down the back of the upper leg, down into the calf, and finally into the foot. This is the largest and longest nerve in the body and is often a cause of pain, which is commonly known as *sciatica.*

Femoral Nerve: The long nerve that runs down the front of the leg is known as the femoral nerve. The sciatic nerve supplies innervation to the muscles at the *back* of the leg and the femoral nerve supplies the muscles at the *front* of the leg. *Pain caused by irritation or compression to the femoral nerve doesn't actually have a name like *Sciatica,* it is just referred to as femoral nerve pain.

Muscles: There are many muscles that connect to the back, and most of them have the role of providing stability to the spine, rather than to provide movement.

Spinal Movers: The erector spinae muscles run from the coccyx all the way up to the cervical spine and form a strong layer of protection to the spine and allow the back to perform the movement of extension (bending backwards). Muscles can often be a source of pain in the back due to the high demand we put on them when we perform lifting activities or when we are in certain positions for a prolonged period of time.

Spinal Stabilizers (Core Muscles): It's very easy to get carried away and go into great detail when it comes to your core, but for the sake of this book, I'll keep it simple. We have our inner core muscles (transversus abdominis, which is your deep core control muscle), outer core muscles (rectus abdominis, i.e. the six pack muscles), and our lateral core muscles (obliques and quadratus lumborum). For an optimally functioning and pain free back, you need all of the components of your core to be strong and working together.

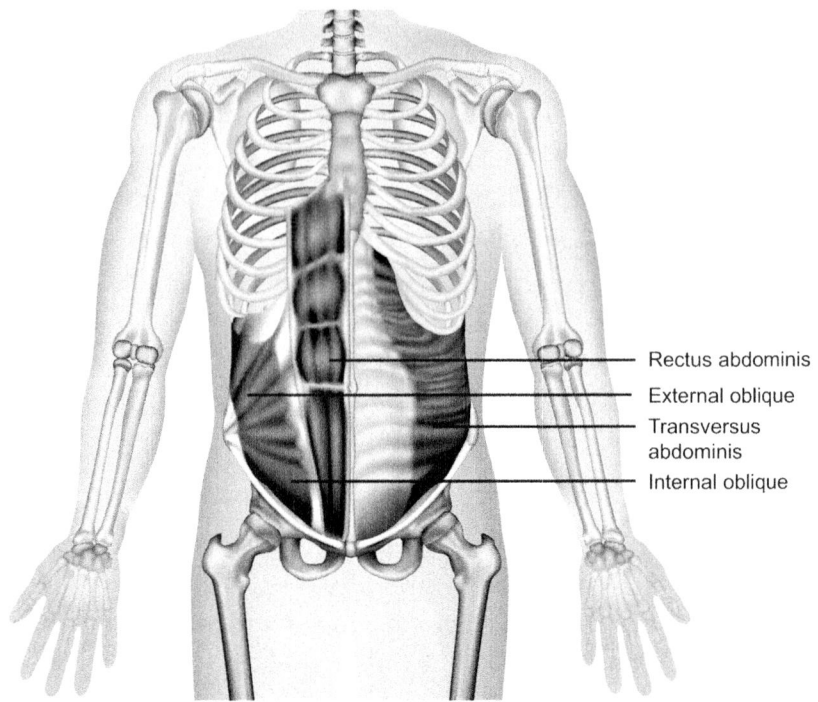

Rectus abdominis
External oblique
Transversus abdominis
Internal oblique

| Spinal Stabilizers

Tendons: A muscle is connected to a bone by a tendon. These strong structures are made up of connective tissue containing high levels of collagen, making them sturdy. The tendons directly in our back actually rarely get injured.

Ligaments: Like tendons, ligaments are also strong fibrous structures, only these ones connect bones to other bones. There are many different ligaments which run up the spinal column. They are frequently a source of pain in the back, due to the high pressure our backs are always under.

MAJOR LOWER BODY MUSCLES

I hope you're feeling a little more clued up about your back now, and if you didn't already, you feel as though you understand the basic terminology. However, when it comes to lower back pain, the focus tends to be solely on the back and not much else is discussed. While this might seem sensible as that is where the pain is presenting itself, the lower extremities can play a key role in maintaining a healthy back. If certain muscles in your legs are either too tight or weak, this can be a reason as to why you have back pain in the first place and might explain why it is not improving with core conditioning alone. Let's go over the main lower leg muscles you need to know about.

Gluteal Muscles: There are 3 muscles that make up your buttocks; the gluteus maximus, gluteus medius and gluteus minimus. The ***gluteus maximus*** is your largest gluteal muscle and is the most visible one on a human body. It actually attaches to the pelvis as well as the sacrum, providing really important support to the lower back region. It commonly is weak in people with back pain but is not often included as part of rehabilitation programs. It has a primary role in walking as it performs the movement of hip extension (taking your leg behind you) and if it's weak when you're walking it can cause your lower back to take more pressure than when your glutes are strong. The ***gluteus medius*** is the next one down in terms of size and sits underneath the maximus, it's another really important muscle for providing stability between your pelvis and your lower back. The ***gluteus minimus*** is the smallest of all the gluteal muscles.

Hamstrings: There are three individual muscles that make up the hamstrings, and these are located at the back of the thigh. They attach from your sitting bone which is called your ischial tuberosity, down to the back of your knee as well. They are often tight in many people with back pain and as they attach to your pelvis this can cause a pulling effect on your pelvis which in turn leads to a pulling on your lower back.

Piriformis Muscle: If you've ever been to a physical therapist or osteopath, you may have heard of the piriformis muscle. It lies under your gluteus maximus and it attaches onto the sacrum (just a bit higher than the gluteus medius) and onto the top part of the outer hip bone known as the greater trochanter. The sciatic nerve often runs through the piriformis muscle or very close to it, and the piriformis is often a culprit for being overly tight meaning it can lead to sciatica symptoms through increased pressure on the sciatic nerve.

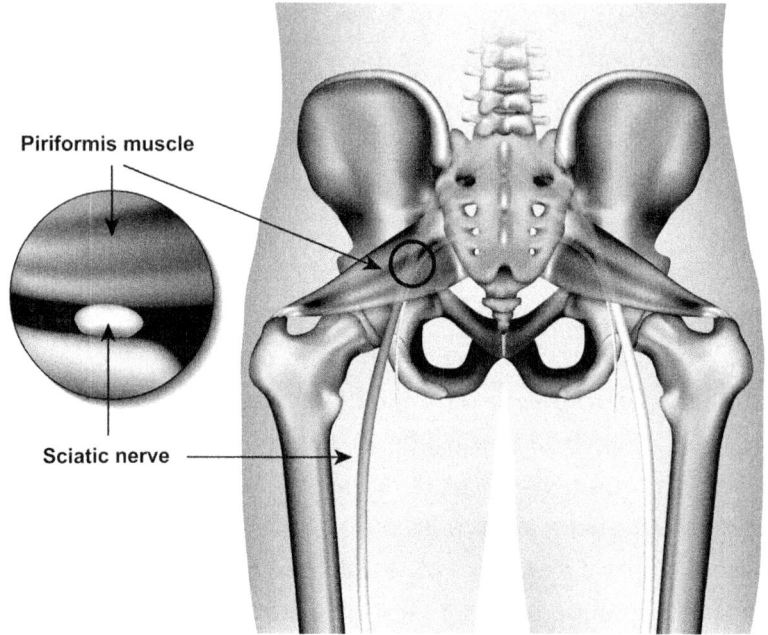

Piriformis muscle

Sciatic nerve

| Piriformis muscle and sciatic nerve

Hip Flexors: The hip flexor muscles sit at the front of the hip region and are, as the name would suggest, responsible for flexing the hip (bringing the knee towards your chest). There are two main hip flexors; the iliopsoas and the rectus femoris. The iliopsoas muscle runs from the lower back to the inside part of the pelvis, and down to the inner portion of the hip bone. Like the hamstring muscles, hip flexors too can become tight causing an increased pull on the lumbar spine, and thus more pressure and pain.

Fascia

Finally, an important aspect of our bodies that play a role in how our bodies function is our connective tissue, otherwise known as *fascia.* This is a part of the body that has largely been ignored for the past several decades, because we have always been more interested in what lies below the fascia, i.e. all of our muscles and organs. The fascia is essentially a layer of tissue that encases our whole entire body, sitting just below the skin. It's continuous, meaning it weaves its way throughout the entire body and doesn't solely sit under the skin–every bone, organ, blood vessel, nerve, and individual cell in our body is enveloped by fascia. Our fascia are the strong woven fibers that create our ligaments, the glass like substance that forms our cornea, and even the material that creates our scars when we injure ourselves. It's hard to put into words exactly how this appears inside our bodies, but it resembles the web of a spider if it were 3-dimensional. I like to think of fascia as a net that is strong and sturdy, yet gentle, sort of holding all of our bones and organs in place as they sway and move.

The fascia is made up of three main components: collagen, elastic fibers, and a fluid matrix. Additionally, the fascia contains nearly six times the amount of nerve fibers as our muscles do, and many of these are interoceptors which give us our sense of physical being. So when we're moving our bodies, and experiencing the world as our bodies do, when we're hungry or feel pain, it's actually our fascial networks that allow us to fully appreciate these sensations. The fascia acts as a tensile network, holding everything in place, while also allowing us to stretch and to move as we please both on a micro and macro level.

Because fascia is interconnected throughout the entire body, when one area is being moved around or tugged, it can affect the fascia in other areas of the body both near and far. Any movements we make cause our fascia to move fluidly to accommodate the new shape our body is trying to form. When you think about the lifestyle of our ancestors, they were constantly on the move in order to survive. Whether they were hunting, walking, running, carrying things, digging, their activities were always variable and their movements were large and taxing. This constant mobility, as you can imagine, kept our ancestors' fascia healthy and strong. Unfortunately today, we are in a world where our activities are limited on a daily basis, and the luxuries of technology that we have created might actually be *hindering* our bodies natural scope of movement.

In the same way that fascial stretching in one area of the body can push and stretch the fascia elsewhere, fascial *restriction* can pull and compress other areas in the body creating *more restriction*. The result of this immobile fascia is a complex web of tension that leads to chronic pain, fatigue, and in some cases, loss of function.

When fascia becomes restricted, dense, and tangled, we feel areas that are painful and stiff. But in addition to the pain, our other bodily systems and structures may be indirectly affected too. This can put unwarranted pressure on our muscles, other organs, joints, nerves, and spine, and thus, create imbalance in our bodies. It almost turns into a vicious cycle of the pain and stiffness causing even more pain and stiffness elsewhere in the body. So how do we fix this?

In order to keep our fascia healthy, we have to remain as mobile and flexible as possible. But this doesn't just mean going for a walk at the end of the work day. I'm talking multi-directional movement, like that you would experience while dancing, swimming, or a full body stretch. It's even recommended that you get up and move around for a few minutes every hour if you work a sedentary job. Our bodies were built to move, and keeping our fascia healthy by doing so, will have a large effect on our overall well-being.

In Chapter 4, I'll go over a couple good stretches for fascia that you can incorporate into your program of choice.

DIFFERENT CONDITIONS

There are many different conditions that can cause back pain, so let's go over some common reasons as to why your back may be hurting. Luckily, the methods for managing them are generally the same, but there are certain specific precautions as well as recommendations for each condition. There are 6 main conditions this book will cover in detail and in the later chapters I'll take you through exactly how to manage each one, so you'll have a specific plan to fit your needs.

The 6 main conditions are:

- Spinal Stenosis (Arthritis)
- Spinal Stenosis (Disc Bulge)
- Spondylolisthesis
- Facet Joint Pain
- Back Strain/Sprains
- General Back Ache

It is highly likely that if you're reading this and have back pain, the reason for your back will fall into one of 6 of these causes.

Spinal Stenosis (Arthritis)

Overview: Stenosis simply means narrowing, so spinal stenosis is narrowing of the spinal column. It is a condition in which there is a narrowing of the spinal foramen (where the spinal cord runs) and/Or the intervertebral foramen (where the nerve roots exit the spine). It is much more common for there to be intervertebral narrowing than spinal narrowing. It is thought to affect anywhere between 250000 and 500000 people in the US alone.

Causes: The most common cause of spinal stenosis in people over 50 is **arthritis**. Where two bones meet, (a joint) there is cartilage that lines the ends of both bones. Arthritis is simply the degeneration of this cartilage, and this can happen to any joint in the body. In the spine, the intervertebral disc loses water content as we age over time causing the vertebral bodies to become closer together. This causes the facet joints (joints between the bones of the spine) to experience increased rubbing due to thinning of the cartilage layer between the bones. This triggers the arthritic process, and the joints start to degenerate. In response to the arthritis, the body attempts to compensate for this by growing more bony parts in the facet joints to provide more stability. These extra bits of bone growth are called osteophytes, and unfortunately these only serve to worsen the problem by narrowing the hollow opening where the nerves exit, which can compress the nerves. An added response of arthritis of the facet joints is that the ligaments attached to the joints thicken (again, to compensate in an attempt to provide added stability). This further reduces the space for the nerves to exit.

Symptoms

Back pain: This interestingly isn't the main symptom associated with spinal stenosis, but occurs when the condition has progressed. It is caused as a result of the arthritis, but also occasionally due to the muscles of the back compensating and becoming overly tight.

Sciatica: When the sciatic nerve which runs down the back of the leg becomes irritated at any point down the leg, this can cause sciatica symptoms down the back of the leg. This usually starts in the buttock and radiates down the back of the leg into the calf.

*If the femoral nerve becomes irritated, pain is felt down the front of the leg. The femoral nerve is much less commonly affected, and this does not have a specific name like that of sciatica.

Numbness: When a nerve gets pinched it can cause other symptoms aside from the pain including numbness, pins and needles, or tingling. The numbness will (like the pain) correlate to which nerve has been affected.

Foot Drop: Once the condition progresses past a certain point then the nerve will have become further compressed and you will notice a weakness in one of both of your feet. Sometimes you may get the feeling of your foot slapping against the floor, or not quite being able to pick your feet up off the ground when walking.

Key clinical signs: Patients with spinal stenosis will notice that their pain is much better when bending forwards compared to bending backwards, and this is one of the key findings I look out for when examining my patients. This is because when we bend forward, the intervertebral foramen (which are small holes in our vertebrae where the nerves exit from the spine) increase in size by about 12%, thus improving symptoms as pressure is released from the nerves. When we lean backwards it reduces by about 20%, worsening the symptoms.

Activities patients will find painful:

- Walking
- Going upstairs or uphill
- Bending backward
- Prolonged standing

Activities that improve symptoms:

- Sitting down
- Bending forward

Spinal Stenosis (Disc Bulge/Herniation)

Overview: A disc bulge is the second most likely cause for spinal stenosis in those aged over 50. As described earlier the disc is made up of a tough outer ring (Annulus fibrosus) with a gel-like inner core (Nucleus fibrosis)–think of it like a jelly doughnut. A disc bulge occurs when the inner core pushes on the outer ring causing it to bulge into the intervertebral space. This can then put increased pressure on the nerve causing nerve pain down the legs.

Spinal disc herniation

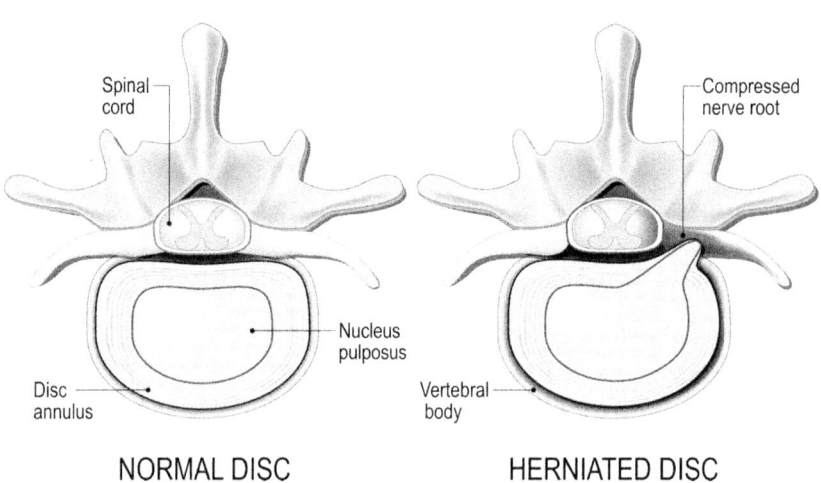

NORMAL DISC   HERNIATED DISC

| Normal disc vs. a herniated disc

Causes: There are two reasons for a disc to bulge–it can either be a traumatic disc bulge or an atraumatic one. A **traumatic** disc bulge is more likely to occur in younger people but can also happen in older adults too. This classically happens with poor lifting technique, or trying to lift something too heavy with a bent back, and it might feel your back gives out on you causing immediate radiating pain down the leg. This would be because the inner core has bulged out against the departing nerve root. This most commonly happens at the lower levels of the spinal (L4/L5/S1). I once had a patient who came in with pain radiating down her leg and a dull back pain on her left hand side. Two days prior, she had lifted a heavy pot while gardening and felt a pop in her back. Afterwards, she had difficulty driving for any length of time, and found it painful bending forwards. This is a classical presentation of a traumatic disc-herniation.

The other type of disc bulge is more common among older adults and that is the **atraumatic** age related disc bulge. As we previously discussed, your discs lose water as you age and this can lead to the inner core becoming more susceptible to bulging back against the outer ring. Atraumatic disc bulges are commonly seen in older adults and are regularly picked up on MRI scans, however we tend not to read too much into the MRI scans unless it matches with the clinical picture (i.e. how you and your symptoms are presenting in clinic).

*Researchers conducted a really interesting study in which they found that 60% of adults aged over the age of 50 had signs of disc bulges on MRI scans with absolutely no symptoms at all. This just goes to show that just because your MRI scan said you have a disc bulge that doesn't necessarily mean this is the root cause of your pain, it may well be there are other factors at play.

Slipped disc? Although it is still used fairly widely, even by medical professionals, I really think it's time to try and phase this old saying out. The reason being is that it creates confusion and also far greater panic for the patient than necessary. The term "slipped disc" would imply that the whole disc has shifted within the spine, and if my patients (or any patients) heard me tell them that they had a slipped disc, this would create immediate panic and the feeling that they shouldn't move their back in case it worsens how much the disc has slipped. The phrase *bulging disc* more accurately describes that only part of the disc moves out of place, which is much less reason to panic.

Symptoms: The symptoms will be much the same as the spinal stenosis caused by arthritis (listed in the previous section), however the activities that improve or exacerbate the pain may vary, as can be seen below.

Key clinical signs: Patients with a disc bulge presentation will typically not enjoy bending forwards at all and this will bring their pain on and find bending backwards to relieve their pain.

Activities patients will find painful:

- Bending forward
- Prolonged sitting
- Driving for too long
- Sneezing/coughing
- Walking

Activities that improve the pain:

- Bending backwards
- Lying down

Spondylolisthesis

Overview: This occurs when there is a slipping of one vertebra on the one below it. This is a fairly common condition in the older populations especially in those aged over 70 and most commonly occurs in the lower back region. It is estimated that between 5-7% of the population have a spondylolisthesis however It doesn't always cause symptoms. The L4/L5 level and the L5/S1 level are by far the most commonly affected levels when it comes to spondylolisthesis.

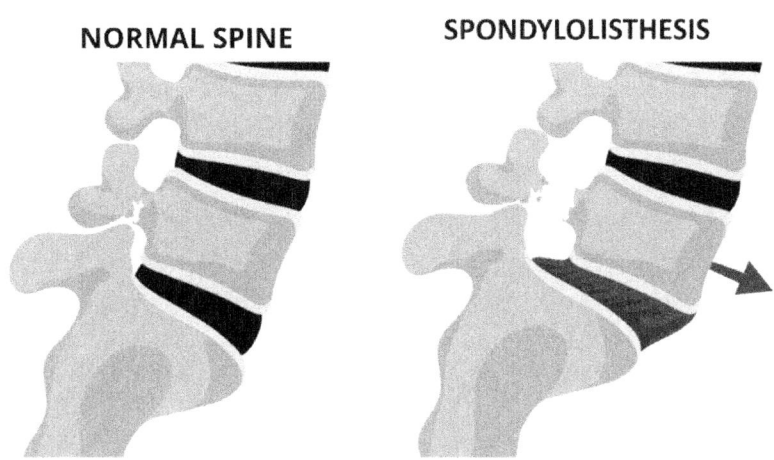

NORMAL SPINE   **SPONDYLOLISTHESIS**

Causes: The most likely cause is the joints in the lower back becoming worn (arthritis) and the stability between the bones therefore being reduced, causing a vertebra to slip. This process is very similar to that of spinal stenosis in the sense that arthritis is at fault, but instead of the foramen narrowing, the vertebra slips forward. This can also be caused by trauma such as a hard fall directly onto your back (this is usually diagnosed by imaging).

Symptoms

Lower back pain: The pain in your back will be from two sources (much like that of spinal stenosis). The first is obviously the arthritis in the facet joints causing the spondylolisthesis and the second is the compensatory muscular reaction where the muscles work extra hard to protect the lumbar spine. The pain will usually be felt in a band across the lower back, with one side being worse than the other.

Sciatica: Pain brought on by irritation to the sciatic nerve by the slippage of the vertebrae. This will be the same as we have previously discussed with pain radiating down the back of the leg. *There can also be femoral nerve pain down the front of the leg, but again, this is not nearly as common.

Numbness, tingling, pins and needles: The pressure on the nerve can cause numbness, tingling or pins and needles.

Foot Drop: This can also occur with spondylolisthesis.

Key Clinical Signs: Patients with spondylolisthesis may present much like that of spinal stenosis in that they don't like bending backwards. This makes sense as the action of bending backwards causes the lower vertebrae to slide forwards.

Activities Patients Will Find Painful:

- Bending backwards
- Standing up from sitting
- Lying/sleeping on their front

Activities Patient Will Find Relieving:

- There are no particular relieving positions but sitting and walking are often tolerated.

Facet Joint Pain

Overview: As explained earlier the facet joints are the small joints in your back running up the entire length of your back, between each spinal bone.

Causes: Facet joints are often injured during sudden movements into extension or rotation–for example, this is a common golfing injury.

Symptoms: The most common symptom is one sided lower back pain which sometimes pinches on a nerve causing a referred leg pain. The most common key sign to look out for a short sharp pain that is provoked by bending backwards or bending to the side that's painful. People will often describe it as a short, sharp pain that comes on immediately upon performing a particular movement that is painful for them.

Back Strain/Sprain

Overview: Back *strain* occurs when the muscles in your back have been overloaded too much either through repetitive injury or a sudden high demand load on them. The muscles might sustain slight mini-tears in them and become inflamed causing pain. A back *sprain* is when the *ligaments* in the back have been overstretched and become painful.

Causes: Repetitive movements such as when gardening or doing the housework is a common form of injury. Sudden heavy lifting without the use of proper lifting technique is another reason as to sustaining a muscular or ligamentous injury.

Symptoms

Lower back pain: This will be the overriding feature of a muscular back pain, this can vary from an intense pain enough to take someone's breath away to a nagging annoying pain which is fairly mild.

Sciatica: If the strain of the muscles are bad enough then there can be irritation to the nerve in the back. This can in some circumstances lead to sciatica symptoms.

Key Clinical Signs: There are three important things to look out for when you suspect there might be a muscular injury. Does it hurt when you stretch it, use it and touch it?

Stretch it: Muscular injuries will cause an increase in pain when the muscle is stretched. So in a back muscular injury it will hurt when you bend forwards. This will cause a pulling feeling in your back.

Use it: The muscles which are likely to be injured are the erector spinae, and they are used when extending the back muscles. Common activities which these are used in are walking, getting up from bending forwards, standing up from sitting. Patients will often describe a stabbing like pain or a short and sharp intense pain, which comes from the muscle being over-used while it is already injured.

Touch it: The final sign to look out for when you feel it may be a muscular injury is whether or not your back muscles hurt when you press on them. If they do, then there is likely some element of muscular source that is causing your symptoms.

*If all 3 of the above are present, then it is likely that at least part of your pain is as a result of the muscles having been injured. Most muscular related pains are usually short lived and can resolve fairly quickly with the right management. With long-standing back pain, you can still get muscular pain usually in what is called a flare up (a short term increase in your symptoms, on top of your baseline level of pain).

A back sprain injury tends to feel a bit deeper than a muscular back strain injury and if those 3 signs mentioned do not fit, then it's likely a sprain injury.

General Back Ache

This is sometimes referred to as mechanical lower back pain but I prefer to simply call it general back ache. A large number of readers will probably fall into this category as it is by far the most common type of back pain I see in clinic. This is stand alone back pain with no symptoms that shoot down into the legs. Arthritis and muscle tension are the two most common causes of general back ache.

Symptoms: Patients will most often describe a pain that spreads across their back on both sides (although it can be on one side only). A deep, achy pain is how most would describe it.

Key Signs: General back ache is often a lot more vague and activities that aggravate it will vary greatly from person to person. But here are some possible triggers of pain:

- Walking
- Lifting
- Cycling
- Prolonged sitting
- Lying in an awkward position

Serious Conditions

For most of you reading this, your back pain won't be a result of a serious underlying pathology. Nonetheless, it's important to understand a few key things to look out for that could be serious, and if you suspect anything suspicious, get yourself checked out right away by a medical professional. Most back pain is mechanical in nature which simply means when you move in a certain way or sit in a position for too long, or lift something too heavy, then your back pain will trigger. A non-mechanical back pain is when there is no apparent trigger to your back pain. If there is a non-mechanical element to your pain, it doesn't always mean there is something sinister going on, but it might be worth getting yourself checked out.

The Key Signs to Watch out for:

Cauda Equina Syndrome: The lower part of the spinal cord is known as the *cauda equina* due to its resemblance to that of a horse's tail. A compression of these nerves is a medical emergency and one that you should seek medical attention for straight away. The symptoms of this include:

- Having a lack of sensation when you're using to the restroom (not knowing when you're bladder or bowels are full or empty)

- Being unable to empty your bladder/bowels, or going uncontrollably due to lack of control
- Sexual dysfunction–inability to get an erection
- No sensation or feeling when you wipe yourself
- Numbness in your saddle region between your legs (inner thighs)
- Having difficulty picking up your feet when you're walking

Other symptoms to look out for:

- Extreme levels of pain: If your pain is resting at a 9-10/10 then I would highly recommend you seek out medical professional advice and not try and attempt the exercises in this book. The exercises may help, however, you should get it checked out first.
- Night pain: If you are waking up at night for no apparent reason with severe back and/or leg pain, then again this is something that should be checked out.
- Sever sciatic or nerve-like symptoms running down *both* legs simultaneously: this is a sign that you may be getting some central cord compression.

*If any of these signs or symptoms are relevant to you then this book will likely not be helpful for you at this stage. You should go and see your doctor to see if they suggest anything, and you might need an onward referral to a back specialist as you may need non-conservative treatment. However, after your pain or symptoms have been reduced, this book will become very relevant for you, to guide you through the rehabilitation process.

Summary

I understand that was a rather heavy chapter and was full of information, but I hope it was helpful. My philosophy is that having a good basic understanding of the anatomy of your back as well as the common conditions which might be causing your back pain puts you at a greater advantage when treating it. If you're at all concerned with any of your symptoms, then I would highly recommend that you seek out medical advice before returning to this book. If you have stand alone back pain with minimal nerve pain down the legs, then this book should be enough to improve your back pain significantly, and hopefully get rid of it altogether.

2

Step 2: Know Your Options

WHEN IT COMES to treatment of lower back pain there is often much confusion with what should and should not be done, as well as what the different health care professionals can offer. Whilst this is not the most important step in managing your back I do still feel it is a key one to have a basic understanding of the varying options that you may have available to you should exercise alone not solve your back pain (Obviously I would dearly hope this book is a sufficient guide for you to manage your back pain, but I'm not foolish to believe that 100% of people reading this will have their back pain resolved).

TREATMENT OPTIONS

Physiotherapy: Physiotherapy (or Physical Therapy in the US) is the profession I belong to. It is a vast profession with many forms and conditions that they cover. Physiotherapists' expertise lies in their rehabilitation capabilities of patients, knowing what exercises to give for what conditions. However, they do also have the skills to provide some forms of "hands-on" treatment. Hands-on treatment refers to the massage, manipulation, and soft tissue release work which can have a great impact on freeing up any tightness in the back region.

Osteopathy: Osteopaths actually work in a fairly similar fashion to physiotherapists but with slightly more emphasis on hands-on work compared to physiotherapists. They are often thought of as "back specialists" as they have a number of really great treatment techniques for the back. As with all hands-on techniques, if there is any tightness of the muscles or stiffness in the joints, then this can be a great place to start.

Chiropractic: The emphasis of chiropractic care is much more focused on hands-on treatment. There is still the element of education, exercises and advice, but not as much as osteopathy or physiotherapy inlcude. All 3 professions work in similar ways in order to reach a common goal, but apply different methods to get there.

Massage/Soft Tissue Work: This is often a treatment technique looked down on by a lot of health care providers, but from my personal experience, it can be a really great tool in treating back pain. It can help to release tight muscles in the back or legs, or stiff joints in the back. This not only has the brilliant effects of providing short term relief to someone's back pain but also usually allows the patients to more easily complete their exercise plan, which is beneficial in the long run.

Massage and soft tissue work would likely not be suitable if you have spondylolisthesis as this could aggravate symptoms. For all the other conditions talked about through this book, these techniques are ok to do.

Acupuncture: Acupuncture has been proven to significantly reduce symptoms in those who have chronic pain. There are two types of acupuncture that you can receive: Eastern and Western. Eastern is the traditional acupuncture which you will be able to get if you go to a traditional Chinese or Asian acupuncturist.

Their philosophy is working to balance the energy systems in your body by placing a sharp, thin needle in certain points of your body to evoke a reaction and relieve pressure. Some people absolutely swear by it and many of my patients have used this in conjunction with a consistent exercise program which drastically improved their back pain. Western acupuncture is a Western medical adaptation to the more established Eastern version. The idea works much the same as massage or soft tissue release work in that an acupuncture needle is placed into or around a painful area or sensitive muscles. This causes a reaction of the muscle/tissue and promotes an inflammatory response promoting healing of the injured site. I am personally trained in this and usually only use this if massage and soft tissue techniques have not worked.

Yoga: Yoga can be a great option in the later stages of rehabilitation when your pain levels are reduced and you can really start to push yourself. It will really work on your core muscles and general strength and flexibility. I would not recommend yoga to anyone with high levels of resting pain or those prone to flare-ups.

Pilates: As a physiotherapist, I am a big believer in pilates-based exercises for managing lower back pain. The emphasis is very much on getting the inner core muscles to work and can be regressed down to very basic levels, as well as progressed to much harder difficulties for those who need it. I am also qualified in teaching pilates to patients, and most back pain sufferers tend to find the exercises very useful in their management plan.

DO I NEED IMAGING?

When people have pain in their backs, the question of whether or not imaging is necessary will pop up at some point for many people. Some might, and some might not need imaging, so in this section we'll go over the things you should consider, and whether or not imaging is necessary for you.

X-rays: There are not many instances in which an X-ray is actually required, or helpful for that matter. If there is suspicion of a fracture (as a result of a fall directly onto your back), then yes an X-ray is absolutely necessary. This will help reveal whether or not you have sustained a fracture (a break is the same thing as a fracture). Apart from this, they're not that useful. It can show arthritis developing in the spine, but an MRI scan will show that better.

CAT/CT Scan: This actually utilizes X-ray technology to build a cross-sectional image of the back. The images produced are more detailed than conventional X-ray images and can reveal bones as well as some soft tissue structures including ligaments, discs or tumors. They are often requested before an MRI scan is performed.

MRI scan: An MRI scan is the gold standard in diagnosis of back pain issues out of all the current diagnostic tools we have, but it too, has its drawbacks. These help show in great detail whether or not you have a disc bulge, where the arthritis is located in your back, or if you have a spondylolisthesis etc. This type of scan is imperative if you are going down the non-conservative route of surgeries or injections. However, what it doesn't do is show you weak or tight muscles which are two of the most important factors to consider when it comes to back pain. Far too often, healthcare professionals base their treatment solely off of the result of an MRI scan. The vast majority of the time if you can address muscle tightness and muscle weaknesses and a few other key areas then you will find your back will take a lot less load and stress and will therefore become less painful.

Blood Tests: While not actually falling under the "scan" category, blood tests are another good option a doctor may consider for you. A blood test can help to diagnose the condition of *Anky-*

losing Spondylitis which is a condition that causes the joints of your back to become very inflamed, stiff, and painful. Your doctor may suspect this condition if you have a significant amount of morning stiffness in your lower back (Sacroiliac joints) lasting more than half an hour after waking, or if you feel generally very fatigued with the pain, and have pain in other joints throughout your body.

DO I NEED SURGERY?

The answer to this daunting question in the majority of cases is, no. Surgery for back pain on its own is rarely advised unless the pain is extremely severe. This is because back pain without leg pain indicates there is no nerve involvement, and it is mainly mechanical pain. Mechanical pain can usually be treated very effectively with the steps outlined later in this book. You can look at posture changes, lifestyle changes, strengthening, stretching, cardiovascular work, and if these all are addressed then the likelihood is that the pain will reduce somewhat, if not entirely. Surgery may go in and scrape away some of the arthritis, but unfortunately, doctors have found that this can actually worsen symptoms by encouraging more arthritis to be triggered after the surgery. Undergoing surgery also won't help with the tightness, weakness or stiffness of the back.

However, if you have exhausted all conservative options and you are still in significant pain with pain radiating down your leg then surgery is certainly an option that you could discuss with your doctor. Below are the following types of surgery you may hear about.

Spinal Fusion: This is the most common type of surgery performed on people's spines. It involves securing two vertebrae together using metal work to give the spine increased stability. This is commonly used in the conditions of spinal stenosis

(Arthritis) and spondylolisthesis but can also be used in cases of a disc bulge. After having a spinal fusion, you will have less movement in your spine because you have had 2 or more vertebrae fused together.

Discectomy: This is when the whole or part of an intervertebral disc is removed. This is done in cases where a disc bulge has been identified and it is pressing on the nerves. The removal of the disc helps to release the pressure off the nerve to stop the sciatic pain down the leg. You might be thinking, "Why, if I have sciatica, would I not just go straight for a surgery?" Well the simple answer is, as good as modern surgical techniques are, there is no guarantee that after having the surgery your leg pain will be cured. For some people it will feel like a miracle after having the surgery, but this is not the case for everyone, so it is usually recommended to try and get on top of disc symptoms using conservative management rather than rushing for surgery right away.

Laminectomy: This type of surgery is where the back part of the vertebrae called the *Lamina* in the spine are removed or shaved down. This is implemented in cases of spinal stenosis as a result of either arthritis or a disc bulge, where there is pressure on the exiting nerve root. A bone graft and metal work (Spinal fusion) is later used to stabilize the vertebrae.

ACUTE VS. CHRONIC BACK PAIN

Acute Back Pain: This type of back pain is usually short lived (under six weeks) and is a short, sudden onset of your back or leg symptoms. You can also experience acute-on-chronic back pain which is when your baseline pain suddenly increases severely. The most likely cause of acute pain is a back strain or sprain as a result of over-doing an activity, or as a result of an injury such as lifting something that is too heavy. This is really important even if you have had back pain for many years and think this doesn't apply to you. Those with chronic lower back pain can still get acute flare ups of increases in their pain and managing it in the correct way is key.

Acute Back Pain Management Plan

1. **Relative rest:** This doesn't mean complete bed rest, as that brings its own problems with it. It just means easing off slightly from your usual routine in order to avoid flare-ups even further. I always advise people to try and keep up with 1 cardiovascular activity, e.g. walking, stationary bike etc., as long as your pain allows for this. If your pain is too severe that you can't even do this you will obviously have to ride out the most severe of your symptoms and as soon as your pain settles then you can begin to get moving.

2. **Anti-inflammatories:** With an acute pain there is very likely to be some inflammation that is driving the pain. Anti-inflammatories like ibuprofen or naproxen help to reduce the inflammation present in an injured tissue, thus reducing pain. People are often tentative about taking medication when their pain is flared up. I always encourage my patients to shift from this mindset. By no means am I saying to go out and stock up on anti-inflammatories, or stronger pain medications for that matter, but I am saying that if your back pain is flaring up, anti-inflammatories can help as long as you use them as directed. If you are unable to take anti-inflammatory medications for any reason, a great natural alternative is *turmeric.* You can

find this in capsule or supplement form in most health stores.

3. **Gentle stretches:** Stretching is important in managing acute pain. The reason we do gentle stretches is so the spine and the muscles don't stiffen up while they're recovering. Stiffening will cause even more problems when the injury has finally healed. When choosing exercises to do during a flare up, you should choose the ones which are comfortable to do. It's important not to do the ones that are painful even if "you feel like they're doing you good." *There are several gentle stretches outlined in Chapter 4–choose any 2-3 of these stretches to do regularly when your back has flared up.

4. **Hot/cold packs:** Now this is a contentious topic and one that no-one has a decisive answer for. I advocate when in a flare up to try to alternate between both hot and cold on the injured area, and if one or the other doesn't seem like it's helping, then phase it out. The heat will allow the muscles to relax whereas the cold will help the inflammation lessen. I would keep the heat on for 10 minutes, somewhere between 3-5 times per day, and a cold pack on for 10 minutes, 3-5 times per day with at least a 15 minute break between hot and cold so you don't shock the body.

5. **Gradual return to normal:** Patients of mine often stick to the initial steps really well and quite quickly can get their initial acute pain down to a normal level fairly quickly. However, where many people tend to trip up is when they are so keen to return to their normal activities, they rush back *too quickly*. The key is, once you start to feel your pain subsiding, think about

increasing the strain on your back by about 5% per day. I thought of this 'rule' a couple of years ago in an attempt to make it easier for patients to visualize small increases in activity levels, and for some reason it just seems to work! I know this is difficult to quantify, but all my patients who I tell this to seem to get it straight away. My point in giving a small percentage number on a daily basis is to encourage you to take it very easy and gradual. This will allow your back to slowly adapt to increased stress on it rather than a sudden and major increase of stress all at once.

Chronic Back Pain: This is when back pain lasts longer than 3 months and is one of the leading causes of disability around the world. Nearly all chronic lower back pain will start off as an acute episode, which for a potential number of reasons, never settled. The most common cause of chronic back pain when you are aged over 50 is arthritis, followed by disc bulges, but any one of the causes we previously discussed can lead to your back symptoms becoming chronic. How we treat chronic lower back pain is the premise of this book, so if you are able to follow all the steps then your back pain should improve significantly, and for some of you, resolve completely.

3

Step 3: Posture and Pain Triggers

WELCOME TO STEP 3! This chapter is very important in managing your back pain and I fully hope that you pick up a useful pointer (or many pointers) that will help to improve your pain. Before we go into the different types of posture and provide you with practical tips on how to improve yours, it's important to first understand the neutral spine.

THE NEUTRAL SPINE

The neutral spine is the most optimal alignment for your back, allowing for the least amount of force through the vertebrae. The vertebrae are evenly stacked on top of each other so the muscles, ligaments, and tendons are not having to be stretched or pulled to keep the spine upright. When we have back pain, it's likely that you are overloading your back in a particular direction and this is triggering your pain. It is possible to keep and maintain a neutral spine throughout most of the day's activities, and that is what this chapter is about. The point of this chapter is not to panic you into thinking you've got to walk around with a stiff straight back

24/7. Your back does need to move and bend, and it is healthy to do so, however, poor repetitive postures can lead to pain over time. Therefore, this chapter is going to educate you on the possible triggers that may be causing your back pain and the practical steps you can take right away to help tackle the problem.

Posture–this word really does get thrown around a lot by pretty much everyone, including health care professionals. But "stand up straight, and keep your shoulders back," seems to be the only pointer that anyone knows when it comes to it. I'll now go over the 4 categories of posture as well as other potential pain triggers, and give you tips on how to alleviate some of the symptoms you may be experiencing in the different positions. Sitting, standing, lying, and walking are the 4 areas we are going to cover in terms of posture categories. Lifting, driving, sneezing, and coughing are 4 other common pain triggers which we will cover. They will not all apply to everyone, and some of the pointers you may already be familiar with, but I hope everyone reading this will pick up at least one useful tip that just might have a positive impact on your back.

SITTING POSTURES

No matter what is causing your back pain, having a good sitting posture is important in keeping your pain under control. Sitting is often cause for discomfort for many with back pain, thanks to the greater lengths of time we all spend sitting down these days. Between the following two suggestions, choose whichever one feels more comfortable to you. If you like them both, there is no reason you can't do both–switch up your seated posture throughout the day if you'd like!

. . .

The 110/90 Sitting Posture

What is it? It sure would sound better if it was the 90/90 posture, but unfortunately, the most optimal position is 110 degrees to 90 degrees. In an ideal sitting posture, your thighs should be angled down slightly to create the 110 degree angle between your hips and your spine as pictured below. Your knees should have a 90 degree angle with both feet placed flat on the floor. This encourages your lumbar spine to come into a more neutral position.

How can I achieve this position? To achieve this position you might need to pop a pillow or two under your bottom or purchase an ergonomic pillow online to create this angle. *Shorter people*—you may need to place a foot stool under your feet. We don't want your feet to just touch the floor as this can over extend the spine.

Why 110/90? The angles don't have to be precise, but try to get as close as you can. The angle encourages your lower back to come into a neutral spine position, and if you're sitting for long periods, you want your spine to endure as little stress as possible.

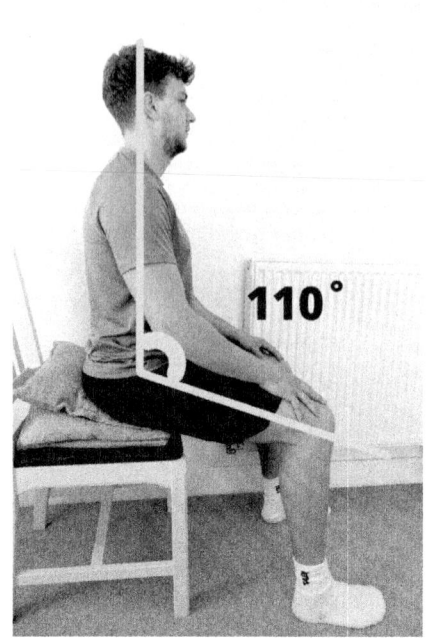

110/90 Sitting Position – the angle between the
back and the thighs should sit at around 110
degrees, while your knees should remain around 90
degrees (these angles do not have to be perfect)

Lumbar Roll

What is it? The use of a lumbar roll, or other form of lumbar
support like a rolled up towel, is a great way to help your back
achieve a neutral spine, especially if sitting aggravates your back
pain. This can be used when sitting at your desk, on the sofa, or
driving your car. You can take one of these with you wherever
you go.

How can I achieve this position? You can use an actual lumbar roll
(which you can buy online), or simply use a rolled up towel
placed behind your back where your arch is. Be careful not to

have the roll too thick, as you want to avoid going too far in the other direction, thus increasing the arch in your back too much.

Why use a lumbar roll? It encourages your back to maintain the natural 'S' curve throughout the spine. When we sit without one, we all know what happens. Our neck and shoulders roll forward making us hunch over, and our lumbar region sinks to find the back of the seat. This might not feel like it's doing much damage when you're just sitting there for 5-10 minutes, but over time it can cause your lower spine to take much more pressure than it otherwise would. When sitting you want your lower back to maintain the arch that it was designed to have. This allows for an even weight distribution throughout the back and into the pelvis, and thus, puts minimal pressure on the back.

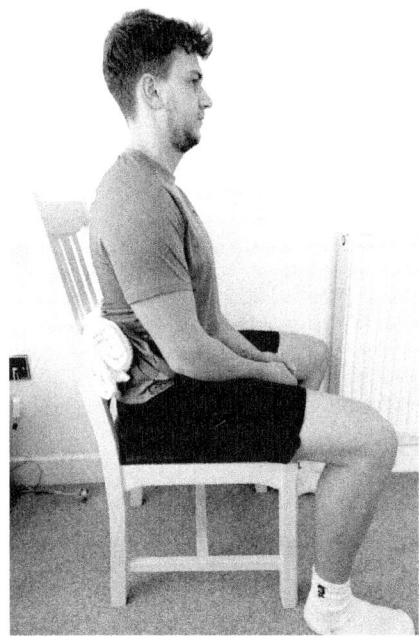

Place a lumbar roll or a rolled up towel as shown, while sitting in chairs that don't provide any support.

Say No to Crossed Legs

What is it? Very simply, this is making a conscious effort to stop sitting cross legged. This might take a lot of mental effort to change if you've been crossing your legs for many years, but I can assure you that avoiding it is an important step in reducing your back pain.

How to achieve this position? This one is the most simple, but arguably the most difficult. If you can, stop sitting cross legged. I often get my patients' other halves to nag at them whenever they catch them sitting cross legged, and hope they quickly give up the habit!

Why not sit cross legged? Sitting with your legs crossed is a habit and not something you just do for 10 minutes once every week. Those who sit this way tend to do it several times per day, every single day, and for the vast majority of people, it's the same leg that's always the "crosser." The act of sitting with one leg crossed over the other causes the hip to rotate outwards and results in the muscles around your hip becoming very tight due to the sustained position. This leads to chronic tightness of the outer hip muscles as well as the hip joint itself, which can then lead to pulling on the back muscles during all of your daily tasks. I promise you, this is a really big one that people often neglect, but is one that can really help for those who do sit cross-legged often.

Regular Breaks From Sitting

What is it? Quite literally, this is just taking regular breaks from sitting positions roughly every 20-30 minutes, in an ideal world. I understand this is a tough ask, and is not always realistic, but if you can aim for this, it will serve your back well. Your break from sitting can be as simple as getting up from the sofa or desk and doing a couple of back bends or side to side rotations, or anything to temporarily loosen up the muscles and joints quickly. Another option is going for a short walk or doing some of the strengthening or stretching exercises we will get onto in the later chapters.

Why do I need regular breaks from sitting? Even if you have followed all the above steps if you don't do this one you run the risk of your back becoming unhappy. As humans, we developed as hunter gatherers and were not designed to be seated in a chair for any prolonged period of time. When we are sitting, there is a 50% increase in pressure on our discs and vertebrae and our back can become tight when we are in a sustained position for a long period of time. Here are some ideas for taking a break from sitting:

- Walking
- Back bends in a standing position
- Lumbar rotations in standing
- Walk up and down the stairs once or twice
- Do some squats or repetitive sit to stands from your chair
- Perform some lying down back stretches (knee hugs, knee rolls, cobra extensions, etc.)

Eye Level Computer Height

What is it? This is very common among office workers but also many of you will have computers at home set up at completely the wrong height for your back/neck. If you're at home and just occasionally using the computer, you may think this isn't a big deal, but every little thing helps and this small adjustment could make a big difference. Your computer screen should be at eye level so you are looking directly ahead at it, and not looking down (or up) at the screen.

How to Achieve this Position? This is a nice, easy fix; buy a stand for your computer or laptop and make sure it is positioned at eye level.

Why does the computer need to be set up in this way? If you are looking down at the computer screen this causes a domino-like effect. First, your head will tilt forwards which will cause your shoulders to become rounded and your upper back arch forwards. This in itself can cause a great deal of neck, shoulder and upper back discomfort. The knock-on effect that this will have on your back, is that your lumbar spine will have no choice but to adapt and lose its arch. This will have the same negative effect that sitting without a lumbar roll behind your back will have.

STANDING POSTURES

Hopefully you've picked up some useful tips on how to improve your posture while sitting. Now, let's discuss the different types of standing postures and useful tips you can implement while standing. So what does an ideal posture look like?

Ideal Posture

- Head: Should be in the neutral position. This means not leaning forward, and ears should be in line with your shoulders.
- Shoulders: Pull your shoulders backwards so they are not in a forward-rounded position.
- Core muscles: These should be engaged to help stabilize your back. To engage your core muscles, gently pull your belly button towards your spine while maintaining your breathing rate.

- Hips: Keep your hips level, and avoid leaning on one side or the other.
- Knees: Should be in line with the bony part on the side of your hip. The knees should be "soft" and not locked when standing. I'll explain this soon!
- Feet: The weight should mainly be concentrated on the balls of your feet.

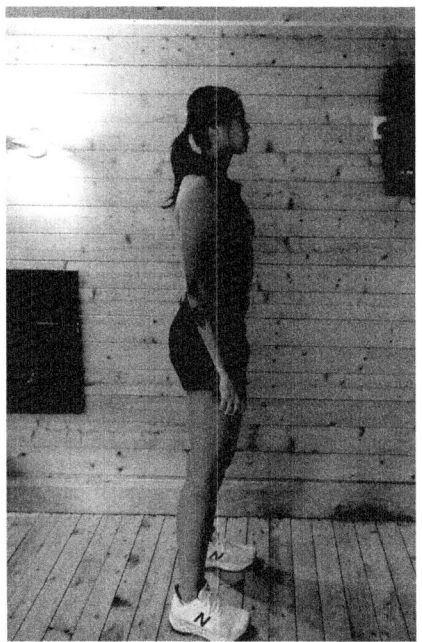

| Ideal posture

*Top Tip: A great way to allow yourself to stand tall with good posture is to take your arms and hold your hands behind your back, as pictured. If you are standing like the photo above, you can simply lock your hands behind your back, and leave them resting over your bottom area.

Now that you know what a *good* posture is, let's discuss the different poor standing postures and, how to overcome these so you are more comfortable when standing.

Flat Back Posture

What is it? This is characterized by the loss of the natural curve in your lumbar spine and the pelvis tilting backwards. The hamstrings will become overly tight, the gluteal muscles will become weak, and the core muscles will become strong. This is a common standing posture among older adults, in part due to the natural wear and tear of the spine causing a natural loss in lumbar spine curvature. However, we can work on a few things to improve this. The best way to see if you might have a flat-back posture is to take your top off and look side-on into a mirror, the key sign is the loss of that lumbar curve which your back should have.

How to correct this posture: Unfortunately, unlike the sitting positions we have previously gone through to correct, certain standing postures are not a quick fix or simple adjustment. It can take time to work on what needs to be addressed. Below are a few things you can do to help with this type of posture.

- **Gluteal muscle strengthening:** Often the hamstrings are tight which causes them to pull on the pelvis, rotating it backwards, and thus flattening the lumbar spine. However, the reason for the tightness in the hamstrings is usually because the gluteal muscles have become weak, causing the hamstrings to compensate and tighten up (see Chapter 5 for gluteal strengthening).
- **Hamstring muscle stretching**: Although the most important factor to address is the weak glutes,

stretching out the tight hamstrings is also important to do (see Chapter 4 for hamstring stretching).

- **Lumbar extension exercises:** With a flat back posture as we have discussed, there is a lack of curve or lack of extension in the lumbar spine. Therefore performing exercises which promote extension is a great option to work on. Examples of lumbar extension exercises include swimming (breaststroke, front crawl), cobra extensions (see Chapter 5), and back bends in standing (see Chapter 5).

Kyphosis Posture

What is it? This might look fairly similar and difficult to distinguish from a flat back posture type. A kyphotic posture is when the upper back is excessively curved and the head sits in front of the shoulders. The shoulders will also be rounded due to the kyphotic posture.

How to Correct this Posture: In people with this posture type, the back muscles will have become very weak, the thoracic spine will have become stiff, and the chest and pectoral muscles will have become tight. This has the impact of the lower back losing its normal arch, putting more pressure at the front of the vertebrae.

- **Thoracic Spine stretching:** The thoracic spine will have become stiff with this type of posture, so in order to correct it, the thoracic spine needs to increase in flexibility. You can choose any of the thoracic spine mobility exercises, depending on what you are able to do. There are not necessarily exercises that are more optimal, but there are simply different options you can try. The most important thing is to get the thoracic spine moving.

- **Back Muscle Strengthening:** The muscles in between your shoulder blades can become very weak if they are constantly on a stretch. If you can train them to become strong, this will help bring your shoulders back and cause a less pronounced thoracic spine kyphosis.
- **Standing Tip:** When standing, you'll most likely notice that your shoulders are rounded forward and your palms are either facing your thighs, or behind you. An easy way to correct this is to turn your palms and have them face forwards. You will feel your shoulders immediately pull back, and that rounded feeling should reduce. Try and remember to stand like this when possible.

See Chapter 5 for thoracic spine stretches and back strengthening exercises.

Locked vs Unlocked Knees

What is it? If you notice that the pain in your back is particularly bad when you stand, it might well be because you are standing with your knees fully locked. When you're standing, your knees shouldn't be fully locked, and if they are, this causes your back muscles to overwork. You can feel this really easily if you place your hands on your back muscles when standing with your knees locked and then soften your knees–you should feel your back muscles relax when you do this. This will allow your legs muscles to take more of the weight and your back muscles take a well earned breather.

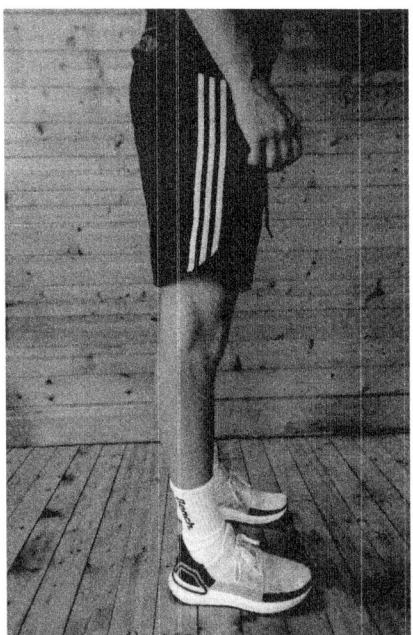

Locked knees (avoid, as this puts increased pressure on the lower back)

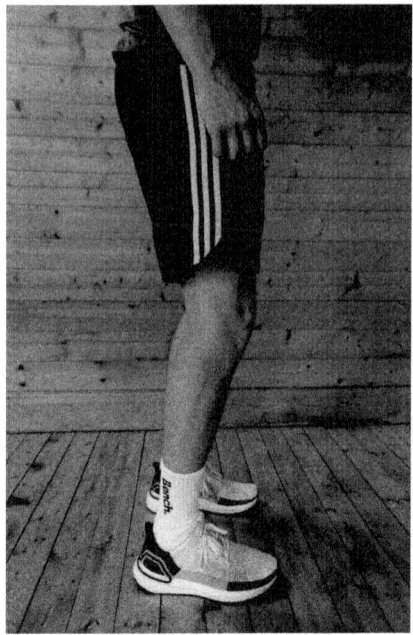

Standing with knees slightly bent takes pressure off the back when standing.

Even Foot Stance

What is it? Now this may seem like common sense and feel fairly trivial, but standing in a symmetrical standing position with your weight spread evenly across both feet is really important for your back. People will often bias when standing leaning onto one leg or the other. While this might feel as though you're relieving pressure on one side at a time and it feels good in the moment, you're actually causing uneven pressure on your back. Over time, this can lead to greater wear on the back and ultimately increase your pain. Your back and your body in general cope much better when both sides of your body take even amounts of pressure. Pain starts to appear when pressure is uneven.

Tip to Standing with Soft Knees: There isn't a great tip other than to make a conscious effort to remember to try and stand with even pressure on both feet. This is another one where you can get your significant other to give you a good nag and a gentle metaphorical nudge every time they see you slip back to your old ways.

WALKING

You might think that you know how to walk considering you've been doing so, pretty successfully, for over 50 years. As with sitting and standing, however, there are certain bad habits you should be aware of when walking that you might not even realize are contributing to your pain. Here is how you can improve your pain when walking.

Lose the Heel-Toe Walk

What is it? Well, it certainly goes against most mainstream teachings of how to walk. The picture below shows the classic idea of how we "should" walk—a strong heel strike when landing, then a transition into a rocking motion on the sole of your foot and finally a strong push forward using your toes. There is much wrong with this way of walking. The heel strike creates a hard shearing force from your heel up through your shin bone, into your knees, and ultimately to your hips and lower back. If this is repeated step after step after step, eventually it will take its toll on the joints in your legs as well as most certainly your back.

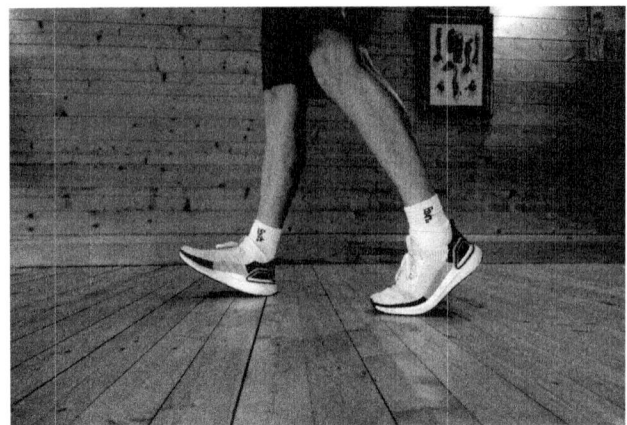

| Example of heel striking that we want to avoid

So how do I walk properly? Well the answer is when you are walking, try and land on your midfoot, not your heel. This forces the calf muscle as well as the quadriceps (thigh) muscle to act as shock absorbers and sends a greatly reduced reaction force into your back. This is similar to how our ancestors would have walked many thousands of years ago and is the preferred technique of walking for our bodies. This might feel a bit odd when you first start walking in this new way, but over time most people end up really enjoying the way they walk. *Note: If you try this for a couple of weeks and you get to the end of 2-3 weeks and you're really not getting along with then don't worry, stop it and try another technique discussed.

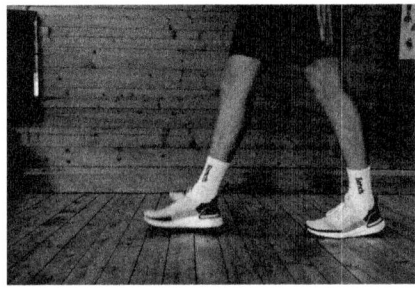

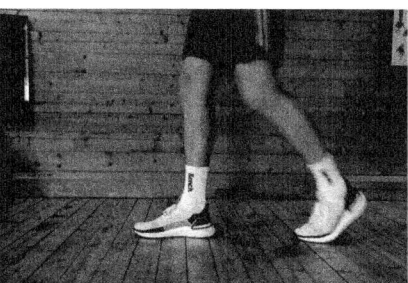

Mid portion of the foot striking ground as opposed to the common heel strike

Walk Faster!

Why Walk faster? A shorter but faster stride length is quite simply better for your back. I can imagine the horror that some of you might well be feeling while reading this, and this won't be appropriate for everyone. Your pain levels might be too high, you may have other conditions stopping you from walking fast, or you may be unsteady on your feet and walking with a stick or cane. But for those of you able to try this, I really hope you will feel what a lot of my patients do when changing to this faster mode of walking. I first learned of this idea 3 years ago when I attended a posture and movement course in London. The following week, I decided to try it out with a few of my patients. I had mixed results then, and still do now, but I would say that around half of my patients find that it improves their back pain, while half find no improvement. Give it a go and see how you find it. The reason this improves some people's back pain when they're walking is that it increases the movement through the pelvis, and therefore, the spine. And we all know by now that the more movement the spine gets, the happier it is.

Top tip for walking faster: Now, I'm not asking you to become an Olympic-grade walker, but just try to reduce your stride length and increase your walking speed by around 10-20%. You can also try swinging your arms more which will give you momentum and will encourage a faster walking pace. This also has the added benefit of increasing thoracic spine (mid-back) rotation, which increases the mobility of your lower back.

Use Your Glutes

Here we are again, back to your glute muscles. If you hadn't realized already, they are really important in improving your back pain, this time for your walking. When we walk, the gluteal muscles are the primary driver for propelling you forward, but most of us have relatively weak glutes when we walk and instead rely on our hip flexors (the muscles at the top of your quads/thighs, just under the hips) to drag your leg forward. You need to change your thought process and focus more on using your glute muscles to push down into the ground, thus sending your leg forward. A good tip to help you start recruiting your gluteal muscles more, is when you're walking, place your hands on the sides of your buttocks and make sure you feel them contract.

Cushioned Insoles

Why walk with cushioned insoles? This works on the same principle as to why we want to avoid walking heel-toe. Having soft cushioned insoles helps to cushion the impact that your ankle, knee, pelvis and lumbar spine take when walking. This should not be confused with a heel raiser–that is not what we want at all, as that can actually lead to other problems.

SLEEPING

Sleeping is often forgotten when it comes to discussing posture but it's arguably one of the most important. You spend approximately 1/3rd of your life asleep, so learning how to sleep well is really, really important. Think about it, if you have a poor sleeping position and you are in that poor position for 8 hours every night, your back over time is going to pay the price. When you're sleeping you want your spine to maintain that neutral alignment we've already talked about.

Stop Sleeping on Your Stomach

Why? Sleeping on your front is by far the worst position you can adopt when you're sleeping–there's no other way to put it. First, when you sleep on your front you need to be able to breathe, and to do this, you usually have to rotate your head sideways. This puts your neck under a significant amount of tension for a prolonged period of time. Second, your stomach isn't well supported when you sleep on your front, causing it to sag into the bed which can tighten up your lower back muscles. This is usually the reason why stomach sleepers wake up with a stiff and tight back in the mornings.

Tips for Back Sleepers

Pillows under legs: Many people are generally tight in their hip flexor muscles (Muscles at the front of your thighs) and when you are sleeping with your legs straight out in front of you on your back this causes a pulling effect on your lower back. Sleeping with pillows under your lower legs is a great way to shorten these hip flexors muscles and reduce that pulling effect. There is also a great tool you can buy called a 'leg elevation pillow' which provides a similar effect to usual pillows but often people find it more comfortable (The height I usually recommend is between 8-12 inches tall).

1 Pillow under head: Far too often I see people sleeping with two pillows under their neck. This promotes a forward flexed neck which can obviously lead to neck pain but also lead to a stiff thoracic spine, and a stiff lower back.

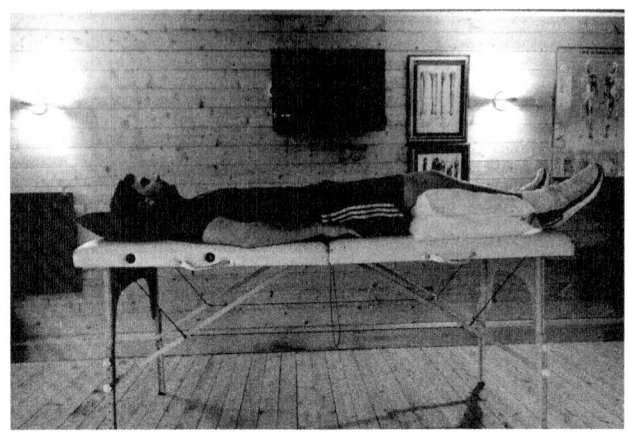

Sleep with one pillow under the head if possible, and prop one or two pillows under your legs to relieve pressure from the lower back

Tips for Side Sleepers

Support under lower back: You can either place a small pillow or a Mckenzie night roll to provide support to your lower back curve. Without a support in place, this can cause your lower back to sag into the bed, losing the neutral spine which the back needs. You may or may not get on with this but it is certainly worth trying.

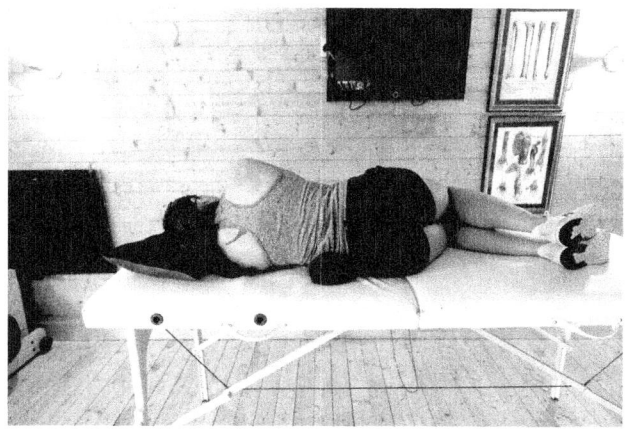

Lumbar roll or rolled up towel used for support when sleeping on your side

Try a pillow in between your knees: This can be a great tip for those waking up with pain on one side of your back. The pain in your back might well be because when you're sleeping on your side this can cause your pelvis to rotate and thus your lower back rotate as well. Once again this deviates the spine from its neutral position.

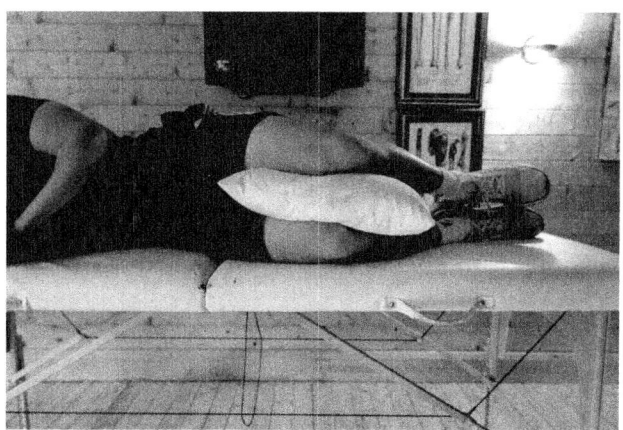

OTHER PAIN TRIGGERS

Bending and Lifting

We all know the importance of bending our knees when we need to lift something heavy. Lifting heavy objects with a curved back is one of the fastest ways to put your back out. It causes very high loads through your lumbar discs pushing the inner core to the back part of the disc, increasing the chance of a disc bulge. Also, simply bending forwards time and time again can also provide the same cumulative effect that lifting heavy objects does. This is why people can often 'put their back out' by doing rather innocuous tasks such as brushing their teeth, bending down to pick a pen off the floor, tying their shoe laces and so on. Learning how to bend properly and lift correctly, could be the most important piece of information you take away from this book. This message is especially relevant to you if you find lumbar flexion (bending forward) is a pain trigger for you. If you have stenosis or spondylolisthesis, I would argue it is still important to know how to do this and practice these tips, but lumbar flexion exercises are key for your program as well.

How to Bend Properly–The Hip Hinge

As humans we bend forward a lot in our modern day lives, much more than our ancestors had to and much more than we should be for our spinal health. It is estimated that we go into lumbar flexion 2000-4000 times per day whereas we bend backwards just a few hundred times. If we are able to reduce the amount of times we ask our back to do this movement and instead train the hips to do the movement for us (which they're designed for) then our backs will accumulate much less strain.

What is a Hip Hinge? The hip hinge encourages the lumbar spine to stay in a neutral position while the movement comes from the hip joints instead. You'll notice when you bend forwards normally, most of the moment comes from the arching of your back and your hips don't produce much movement.

Hip Hinge for Minimal Bending

1. Stand in an upright position with your feet hip width apart.
2. Place your hands on the front of your thighs.
3. Make sure your spine is in neutral and gently pull your shoulder blades together.
4. To initiate the hip hinge, push your bottom backwards and run your hands down the front of your thighs until your hands reach just above your thighs (this will feel a bit like a squat). *Imagine you're in the shortstop position in baseball.
5. You will have noticed that you were able to bend down without directly bending your back.
6. To return to the starting position, squeeze your bottom muscles and bring your hips up and forwards; your back will stay in that neutral spine throughout the movement.
7. You can use this technique to lift heavier objects. When you have performed the hip hinge and partial squat place both hands on the object to be lifted. Hold the object tight, making sure to fully engage your arm, chest and core muscles. Then return to the starting position by squeezing your gluteal muscles and driving up, leading with your hips.

Practice how to hip hinge regularly and over time the movement will become second nature. This can be used for everyday tasks; brushing your teeth, washing up, going to sit down on a chair. If you learn to focus the movement in terms of a hip hinge instead of a lumbar spine movement you'll soon notice the benefit.

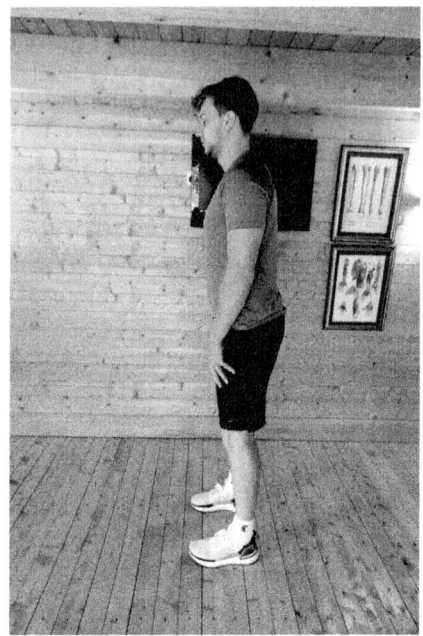

Starting position before a hip hinge

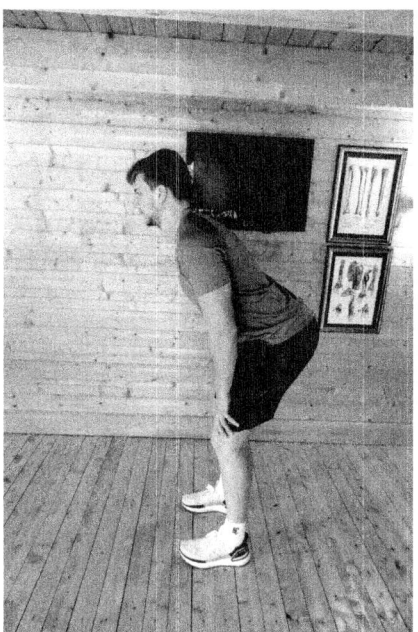

Full hip hinge – Bottom sticking out while the back
stays straight

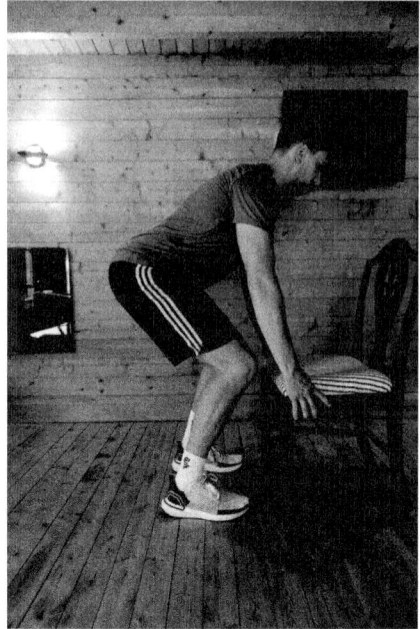

Using the Hip Hinge to lift an object which is hip to knee level

Hip Hinging for Getting Lower

So what should you do if you need to pick something up closer to the ground or off the floor such as a pen? Well you can still use the hip hinge technique but using a lunge movement instead. There are two options; Hinge and lunge or single leg hinge using support. You can try both and decide which one you prefer. For those with dodgy knees the single leg hinge using a support will likely be the better option for you.

Hinge and Lunge

1. Start in a step-stance position with one leg behind the other and slightly out to the side.
2. Perform the hip hinge you have previously learnt. Push your bottom backwards while keeping a lovely neutral spine.
3. From here perform a lunge down to the ground taking your weight predominantly through your right leg while maintaining the hip hinge position.
4. To come back from this position, push your front foot firmly into the ground and squeeze your bottom muscle. Come up by bringing your hip upwards and forwards while contracting your bottom muscle.
5. *You should think about the return phase being a hip movement and allowing the back to follow naturally.

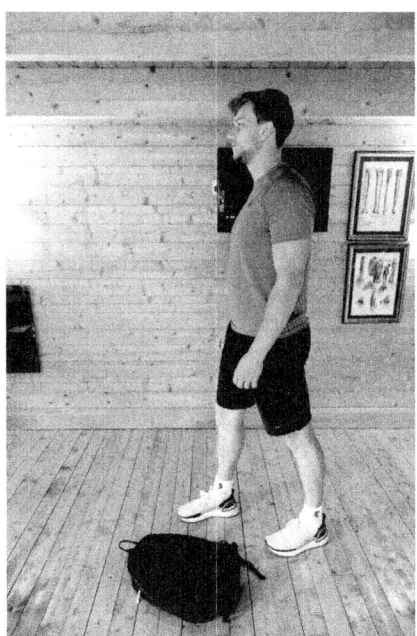

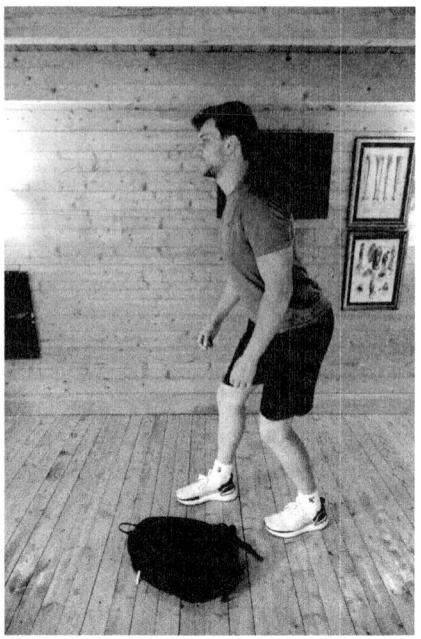

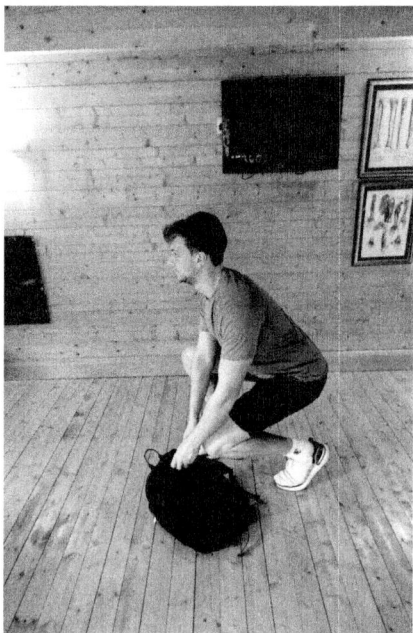

Hinging and lunging to pick objects up off the ground

Single Leg Hinge Using Support

1. Have the support (whether it be a chair, table, desk) by your side and stand in a step-stance position again.
2. Initiate the hip hinge by driving your bottom backwards while maintaining the neutral spine.
3. Take your leg closest to the support off the ground leaving your leg furthest away still in contact and still in the hinged position.
4. From here maintain the hip hinge position with a neutral spine and you bend further from your hip and your knee to lower yourself to the floor.
5. To return from this position, engage your bottom muscles and drive your hip up and forward.
6. *You can lift heavier objects using this technique as well. Once you are down at the bottom of the movement, hold the object you want to move in your hand. To return to the starting position you need to push through your arm which is in contact with the stable surface while at the same time doing what you did beforehand (contract your bottom muscles and drive up using the hips to initiate the movement). This will concentrate the pressure through your arm and stationary leg and not through your lower back.

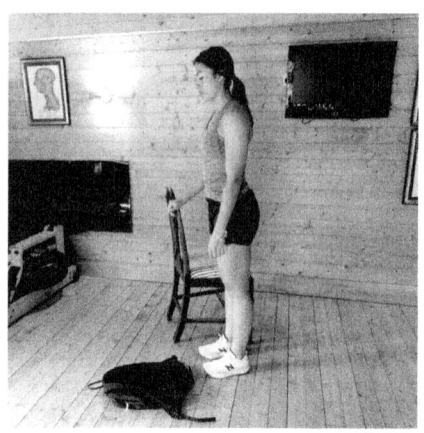

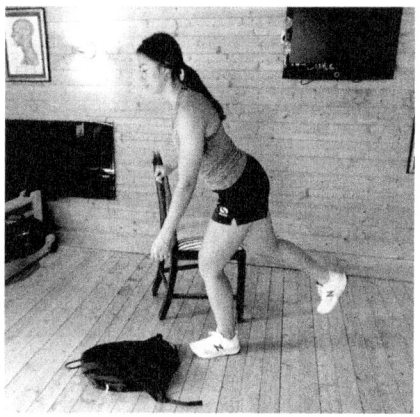

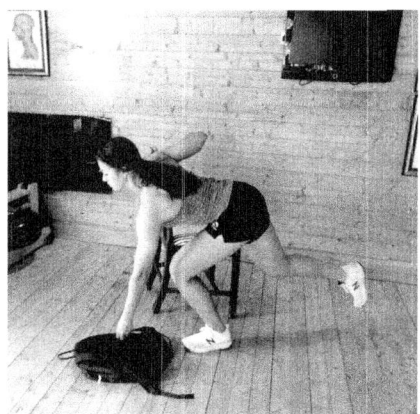

Single leg Hinge using support approach to the ground. Back is in a neutral spine and the movement is coming from the hip and knee.

Use a Picker

If you are unable to bend or lift using the three techniques just described, due to high levels or pain, for example if your back is in a flare-up, then a good temporary solution is to invest in a litter picker. You can use this to pick up light objects from the floor in order to avoid bending while your pain is still severe. This is obviously not a long-term solution, but will protect your back in the short-term.

Sneezing and Coughing

I'm sure many of you reading this will have experienced the dagger-like pain to your lower back caused by a fierce sneeze or cough. Now, there is really only one cause for this, and that's a disc bulge. However, contrary to what you may think, it's not actually the sneeze or cough itself which causes the sharp pain, it's how you sneeze or cough. Most of us perform these two 'activities' by our bodies curling into a 'C' shape before forcefully contracting our abdominals causing a high amount of force to go through our discs. An amazing technique to prevent this happening in 99% of cases, is to look up when you need to sneeze or cough. This will keep your back in a neutral position and doesn't allow for a high amount of force to go to the front of the discs, greatly reducing the chance of an acute disc bulge.

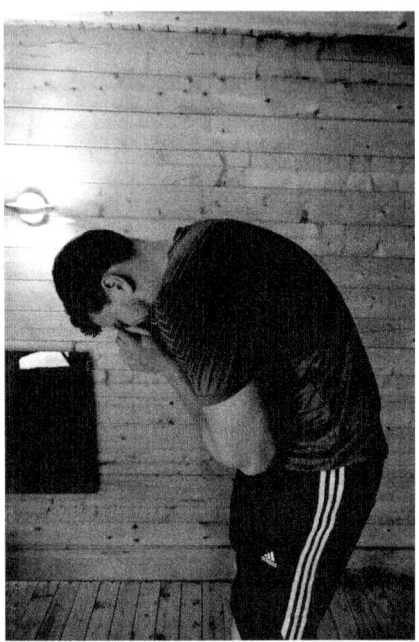

Sneezing in a bent over position puts a great amount of force through your lumbar discs, similar to that when lifting.

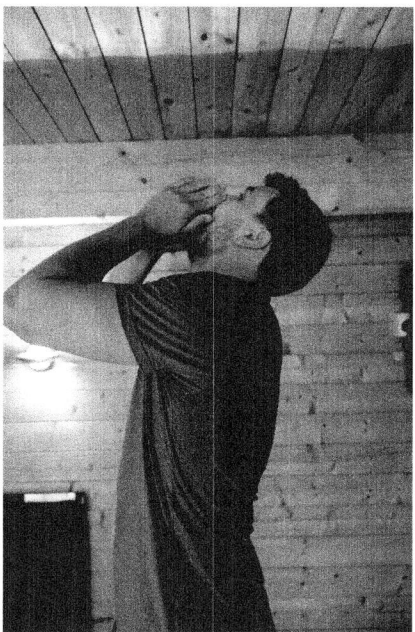

Sneezing in an upright position puts much less force through your discs.

Driving

There are 3 main points to consider if you are getting pain when driving:

- *Low car seat*: Many cars have very low and deep seats, causing the pelvis to rotate backwards significantly thus causing the spine to flatten and lose its natural curve. Place a couple of pillows under your bottom until you are in the ideal sitting position previously discussed (110/90 degree rule)
- *Long drives*: There is only 1 real solution for this and that is to take regular breaks from driving, get out of your car and do some stretches or go for a walk.

- *Use a lumbar roll*: Using a lumbar support in the form of a roll or a rolled up towel is advised. As previously discussed in the sitting posture section, maintaining the natural curve in your spine when sitting is important and one which the lumbar roll will help assist.

That wraps up postures and pain triggers! I hope you've picked up some practical tips that you'll be able to implement to help with your back. In the next chapter, we'll go through stretches that can help manage your pain.

4

Step 4: Stretching

STRETCHING IS a key component of any back pain management program. The muscles, joints, ligaments, tendons, and fascia need to have adequate elasticity and should be as free from tightness as possible for your back to remain healthy. However, I have seen too many exercise routines for people with back pain, and the vast majority of the exercise routine are stretches alone. This quite simply won't work. Stretching alone won't take your back very far—it is just one piece of the puzzle, but it is an important one.

FASCIA STRETCHES

An essential part of my back pain management exercise program is doing lower back fascia stretches at least every morning and evening. The exercises are really simple and are focused on the multi-directional movement of your back. You can choose either one of these exercises or alternate which ones you do, it really doesn't matter. They haven't got specific names but here they are. *They are much easier to follow when you see them actively being performed and instructed, so be sure to check out the free videos I've put together. The instructions of how to access them are at the beginning and the end of the book.

Fascia Stretch #1

1. Stand with your feet shoulder width apart.
2. Hold your right wrist with your left hand.
3. Put your arms out in front of you at roughly head height and rotate in a nice big circle to the left side of your body, pulsing backwards and forwards. Provide a slight pull on your right arm to emphasize the stretch.
4. Do 10 to the left side and then switch hands and do 10 to the right side.
5. Repeat 10 more on each side (2 sets), three times every day.

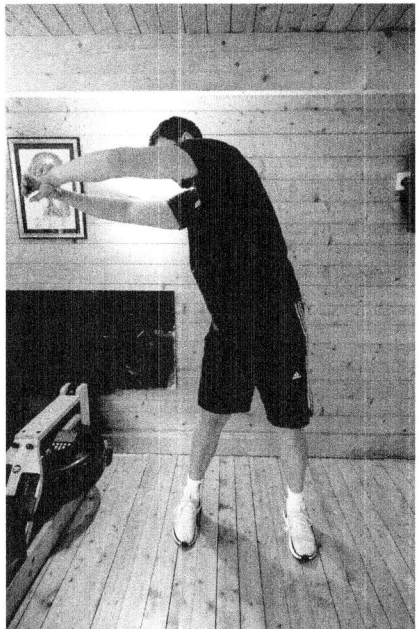

Fascia stretch #1 – hold wrist and pull body in one direction

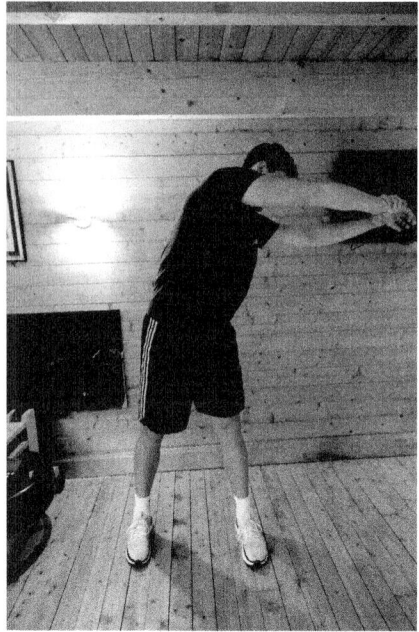

Fascia stretch #1 – switch arms and pull the body in the other direction

Fascia Stretch #2

1. Stand with your feet shoulder width apart.
2. Lunge forward with one leg, and raise both arms in the air above your head. Hold in this positions for 1-2 seconds.
3. Return to the starting position and perform the motion again, 5 times.
4. Once you have done 5 on one side, switch to the other side and perform the stretch 5 more times.

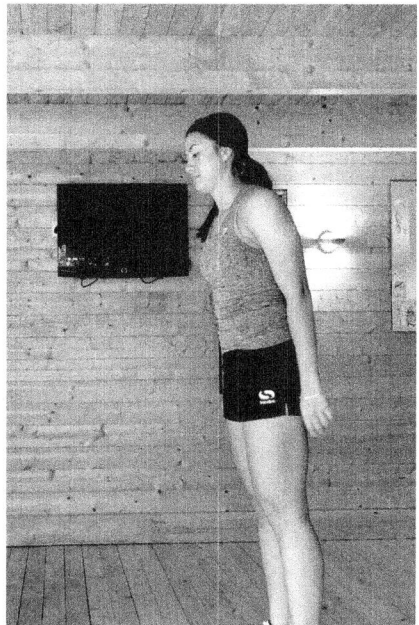

Fascia stretch #2 – starting position.

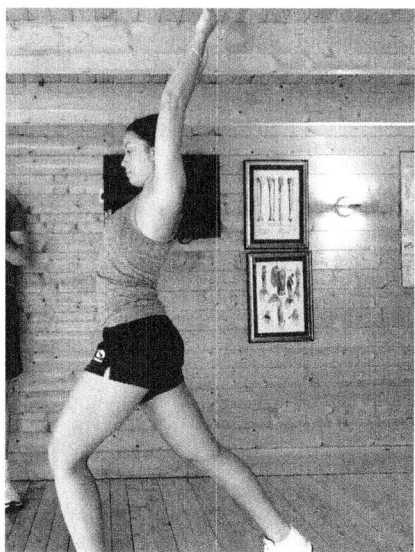

Fascia stretch #2 – final position, hold 1-2 seconds before returning to the starting position to go again.

BODY STRETCHES

For all the stretching exercises we are about to go through, there are 3 levels for each movement or muscle we are trying to stretch–easy, moderate, and advanced. You can try out each one and determine which level is best suited for you. There are 6 stretches in total. I want you to pick 5 of them, choosing between either a lumbar *flexion* stretch and a lumbar *extension* stretch for your program. *If your back is made worse by bending forward, then pick one of the lumbar extension exercises. If your pain is brought on by bending backwards, then pick one of the lumbar flexion exercises. If both movements are painful then pick whichever one feels better for your back.

The levels for all 5 of your exercises can be different for each one e.g. just because you can only do the easy level for the lumbar rotation stretch, doesn't mean you have to stick to the easy level for all the stretches.

Lumbar Extension Stretches

Easy Level Standing Lumbar Extension

This is a great exercise for those of you with general back pain who spend long periods sitting down, as it exercises the back in the opposite direction. It's highly recommended for people with disc bulges, if symptoms are not severe.

**This is not advised for those with spondylolisthesis and if you have spinal stenosis secondary of arthritis, you should think about choosing a lumbar flexion stretch instead.

1. Start in a standing position with your feet shoulder width apart to provide a solid base of support.
2. Place your hands on your bottom cheeks.
3. Arch your back, backwards to perform the stretch into extension.
4. Go as far as is comfortable so you feel a nice stretch across your lower back. Be careful not to push it too far.
5. Hold for 1 second, then return to the starting position.
6. Aim for 10 repetitions. Then break (45 second). Then repeat 10 more, then break and a final set of 10 reps (That is 10 reps X 3 sets).

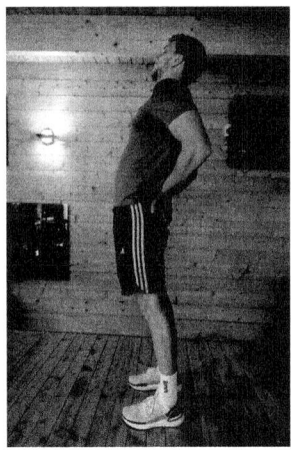

Standing lumbar extension with
hands placed on bottom

Pointers: There is not much that can go wrong with this exercise as it is fairly gentle and shouldn't cause many problems, however, I do occasionally hear. *"It hurts when I go back too far."* The answer to this is fairly straightforward–don't go back as far. If you haven't done this exercise before and you try to go really far back, then your back probably won't like it as it's not used to that position before. Start off with really small ranges of motion and slowly increase as your back gets used to it. Below you can see what conditions it is appropriate for.

- Spinal Stenosis (Arthritis): No
- Spinal Stenosis (Disc Bulge): Yes
- Spondylolisthesis: No
- Facet Joint Pain: No
- Back Strain/Sprain: Try and see
- General Back Ache: Try and see

Moderate Level Cobra Extension on Forearms

The moderate and advanced exercises are almost the same, with the range of motion achieved being slightly less for this moderate stretch. You might have seen it before, it is sometimes known as the Mckenzie extension named after Bob Mckenzie who revealed the wonders it achieved for patients suffering with intervertebral disc pain. This can be done on the bed or even better on the floor. You might think this exercise and the previous standing exercise look very similar. I prefer the cobra extension because the back muscles are relaxed when you are lying down and by pushing with your forearms this allows for a greater stretch of the lumbar spine. The same advice in relation to spondylolithesis and stenosis applies here.

1. The starting position is lying flat on the floor or your bed.
2. Place your forearms by your side with your palms facing down.
3. Perform the half cobra extension by pushing through your forearms and bringing your shoulders off the floor and away from your hands. This will cause your back to arch up.
4. Try and keep your back muscles relaxed if you can.
5. Only go as high as is shown in the picture and hold for 1 seconds, then return to the starting position.
6. Repeat 10 times. Then rest for 30-45 seconds. Then repeat 10 more repetitions and a final 10 more repetitions.

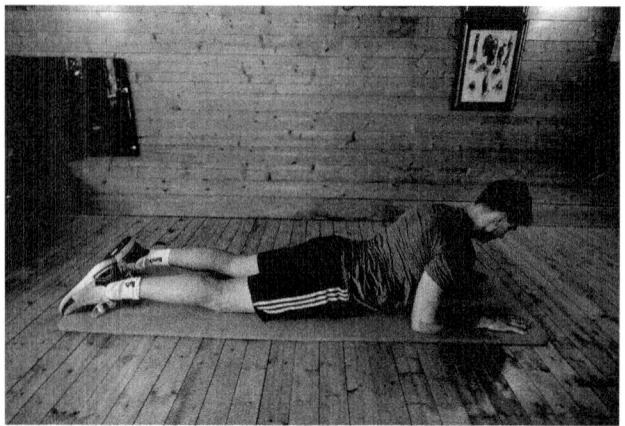

| Half cobra extension to forearms.

Pointers: The key thing with the cobra extension is to try and relax the back muscles when you are performing the exercise and just try and focus on pushing through your forearms and arms.

*Same advice as above in regards to what problems are appropriate for and not.

Advanced Level Full Cobra Extension

This is the same exercise as the *cobra extension to forearm*, however this time you'll be extending your arms much more to achieve a greater stretch of your back. If you felt as though the moderate level exercise was too easy and you didn't feel as though it was doing anything then try this harder version.

1. Adopt the same starting position as before; lie on your front with your forearms and palms flat on the floor/bed.
2. Push up from the floor with your hands but this time fully extend your arms so your back goes through a full extension.
3. Remember to keep your pelvis in contact with the

ground at all times. If it comes off you're losing how much stretch the back receives.

4. Again hold for 1 seconds and then return to the starting position.

5. Repeat 10 times. Rest for 30-45 seconds seconds. Then repeat 10 more repetitions and a final

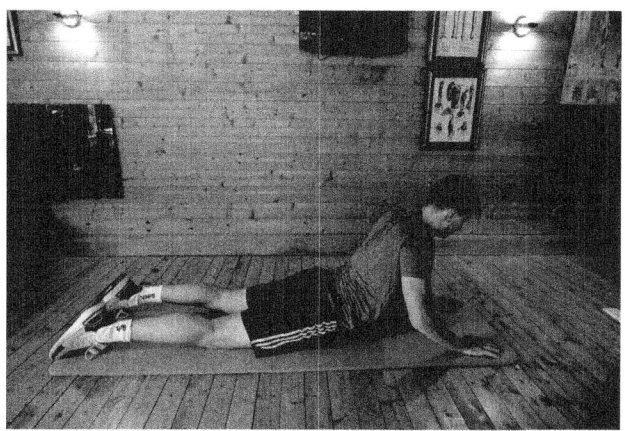

| Full cobra extension with full extension of arms

Pointers: The same advice goes for the full cobra extension as the previous half cobra extensions. Be careful when performing this exercise not to push up too high and don't go into pain.

*Same advice as above in regards to what problems this is appropriate for.

Lumbar Flexion Stretches

Easy Level Seated Lumbar Spine Flexion

Stretches working into flexion are going to be preferable for those suffering with spinal stenosis (arthritis) and spondylolisthesis. A disc bulge will likely not respond very well to lumbar flexion stretches, so probably best to avoid this stretch if that is what's causing your pain. The seated lumbar flexion stretch is a really good one for opening up the lumbar spine, but as a word of warning, if you have low blood pressure, the leaning forward motion may make you feel light headed.

1. Start seated in a chair with your legs just slightly wider than shoulder width apart.
2. To perform the exercise, simply run your hands down the front of your shin bones until you can feel a nice stretch across your back.
3. You can either hold this position for 15-30 seconds and repeat this twice, with a 30 second break in between.

You can do the above method, or you can do the following.

1. Once you get down your shin bones as far as you can, return to the starting position and repeat this repetitive movement 10 times. Then have a 30 second break and repeat again.
2. Either way is fine to perform this exercise, see which one you get on best with.

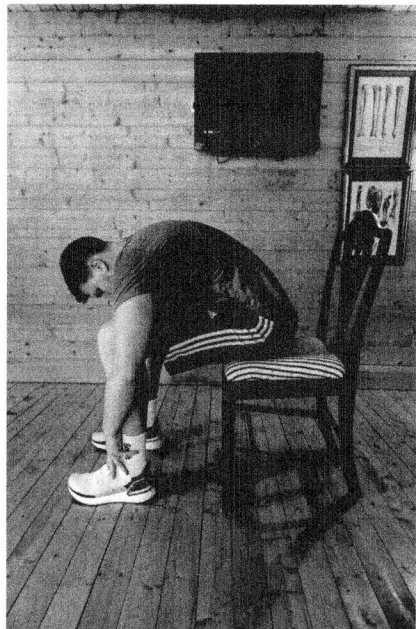

Seated lumbar flexion – run your hands over the top of your knees and down your shins to as far as is comfortable.

Here's what you can use lumbar flexion stretches for:

- Spinal Stenosis (Arthritis): Yes
- Spinal Stenosis (Disc Bulge): No
- Spondylolisthesis: Yes
- Facet Joint Pain: Yes
- Back Strain/Sprain: Try and see
- General Back Ache: Try and see

Moderate Level Supine Dynamic Knee Hugs

The lying down knee hugs are another exercise which is very recognisable in the physiotherapy world. In truth it is probably around the same difficulty level as the seated lumbar flexion stretch. Try both of them and see which one you prefer. It remains a very good exercise at releasing muscular back tension in the lower back region.

1. Start by lying on your back.
2. Hug both knees to your chest using both your arms to hug your knees.
3. Pull your knees close to your chest until you can feel a nice gentle pull in your lower back.
4. Hold the stretch for between 30 seconds, then relax for 30 seconds and repeat for another 30 seconds.

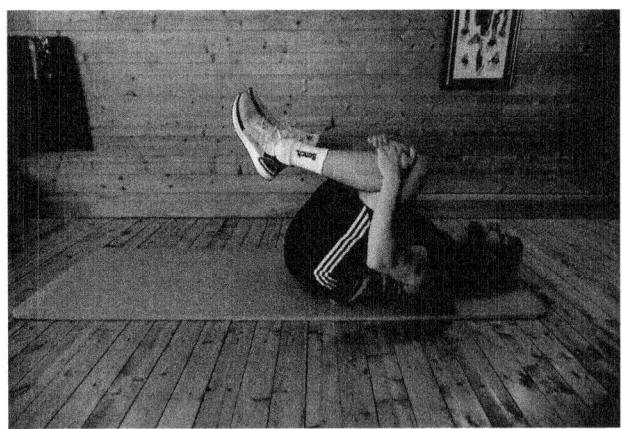

Knee hugs lying on your back. Bring your knees towards your chest and hold for 30 seconds

Pointers: You can try doing a single leg knee hug if you find the double leg knee hug painful on your back. Simply hug one knee to your chest with your other one remaining down.

. . .

Advanced Level Child's Pose Stretch

This is a classic pilates and yoga stretch and it gives the greatest lumbar flexion stretch, if you are able to do it. You will however, find this exercise difficult if you have painful or restricted knees. Achieving great lumbar flexion is vitally important for your everyday functioning which involves bending of the spine. The stiffer your lumbar spine is, the higher chance you have of injuring your back.

1. Start in a kneeling position on the floor, not to be done on the bed.
2. To perform the exercise, drop your heels towards your bottom as far as you can and at the same time reach forward with your arms.
3. Try to reach as far forward with your hands as you can while maintaining your bottom as close to your heels as possible.
4. You feel a nice stretch in your lower back and into your upper back as well.
5. Hold this position for between 20-30 seconds and then relax to the starting position.
6. You can repeat this either once or twice more (2-3 sets in total).

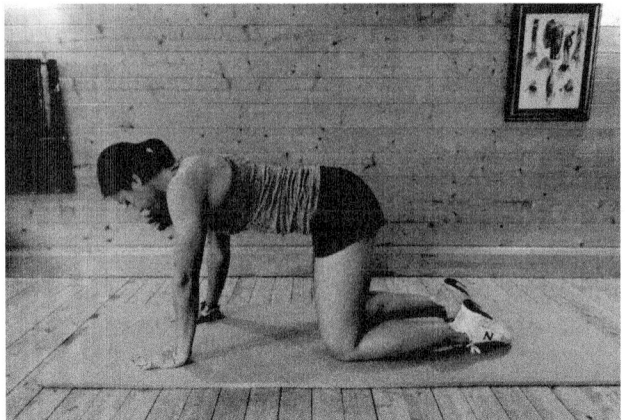

| Starting position for child's pose

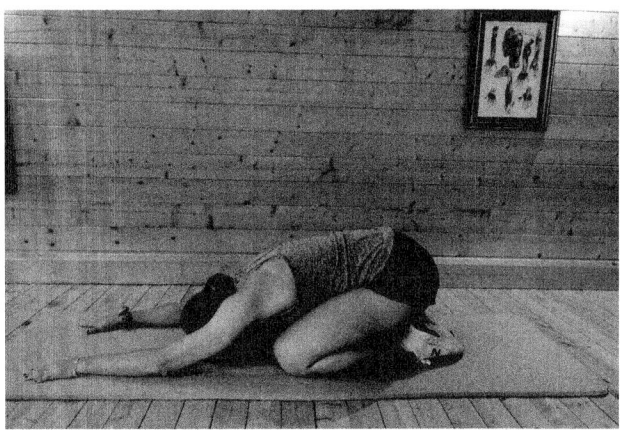

| Child's pose full stretch

Pointers: Remember to take your bottom back to your heel first and then reach forwards with your hands.

Lumbar Rotation Stretches

Easy Level Seated Lumbar Rotation Rolls

The best way to achieve some great lumbar spine rotation is by performing lying down rotation exercises. However, they can be a bit more tricky to do if you're particularly stiff or are in high pain levels. This seated rotation stretch actually works both thoracic spine (mid back) rotation as well as lumbar rotation. There's no specific conditions which shouldn't be able to perform this exercise, however as with all exercises if you feel though it's making your pain worse, then stop.

1. Sit up tall in a chair with your back not resting against the back of the chair.
2. Have your arms out to the side of you in the chicken wing position.
3. Now rotate your body from side to side trying to get your chest to rotate as far round to one way as possible.
4. When you reach as far as you can then return to the starting position and immediately rotate your body to the other way.
5. Continuously do this movement for 10 repetitions each way with a 1 second pause to each direction. Have a 30 second break and perform 10 more repetitions to each direction. You can do this one more time if you find it useful.

*This can be used for all conditions.

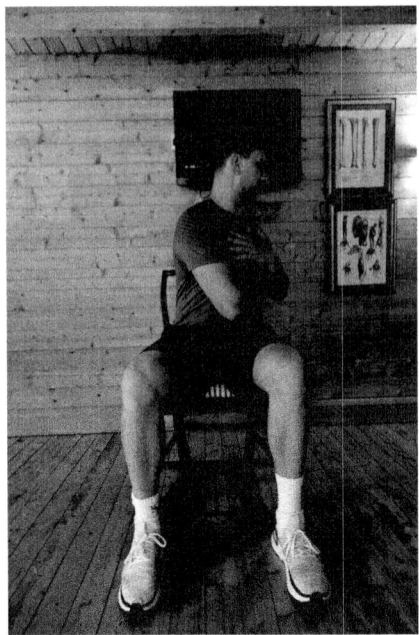

Lumbar rotation whilst sitting with arms crossed across your chest.

Pointers: Remember to sit up nice and tall when doing these exercises and try not to slouch. Slouching will put your lumbar spine in a poor posture and limit the amount of rotation you're able to achieve.

Moderate Level Supine Knee Rolls

This exercise is widely used in the physiotherapy world and for good reason. It is a brilliant exercise and promotes good lumbar spine rotation. It can be a great exercise to do if you're having a flare up of pain as it can help relax tight muscles and joints in the lower back region. In our modern day lives, our spines tend to get exposed to minimal rotational movements throughout the day.

1. Start by lying on your back with your knees bent to 90 degrees as shown.
2. Keep your feet and knees together and place your hands just away from your side, face down to act as a good support base.
3. Gently take both knees to one side dropping them as far as is comfortable for your back.
4. Hold the position for just 1 second and then return to the starting position and then take your knees to the other side.
5. Repeat this movement from side to side for between 30-45 seconds. Then have a break and repeat once more.

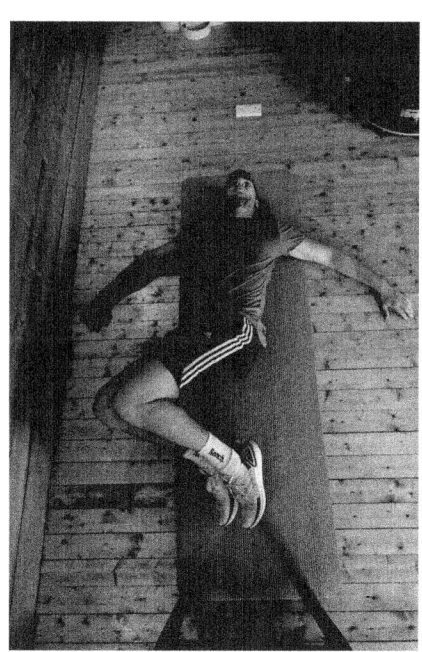

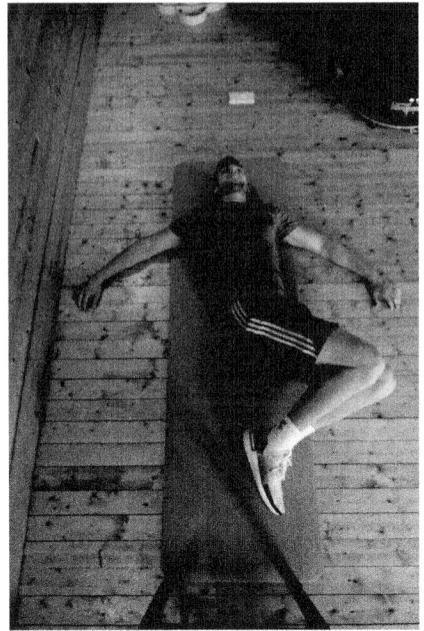

| Lying knee rolls from left to right side

Pointers: Some people, if their back is very stiff, find it gets painful when they take their knees all the way to the floor. As your spine gets more supple this problem will be reduced, however in the meantime you don't need to go all the way down, just do smaller ranges of movement of the knees and over time slowly increase this until you can get them all the way down.

Advanced Level Lying Lumbar Rotation

This lying lumbar rotation stretch is quite a bit more challenging for the back so it won't be for everyone. However, for those of you who can tolerate it, it will work wonders for your back. It allows the lower back to achieve maximum rotation.

Improving your rotation will in turn improve your flexion movements, extension movements and generally make your back feel
much more free.

1. Start by lying on your back (can be done on either
   your bed or floor) with your right arm out at shoulder
   height and your right leg bent to 90 degrees.
2. Throughout the movement you are wanting to keep
   your right shoulder in contact with the floor.
3. Bring your right knee towards your chest.
4. With your left hand pull your right knee down
   towards the floor
5. Only go as far as you are able to. Don't push into the
   pain, just go to the strain.
6. You may feel it either in your lower back or your
   gluteal muscle, either is fine.
7. Hold for 30 seconds at a time and repeat on both
   sides, then break for 30 seconds and repeat two
   further sets.

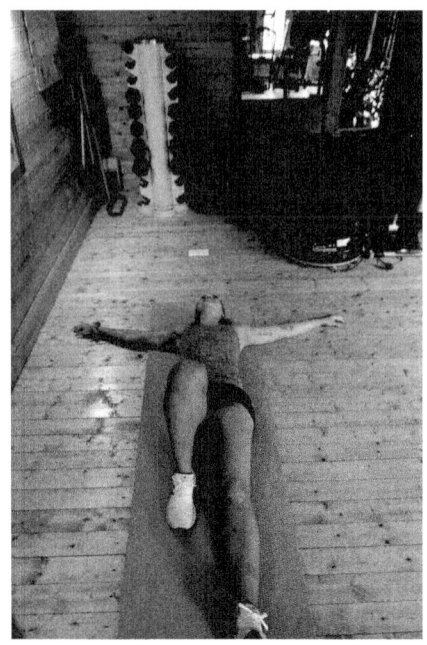

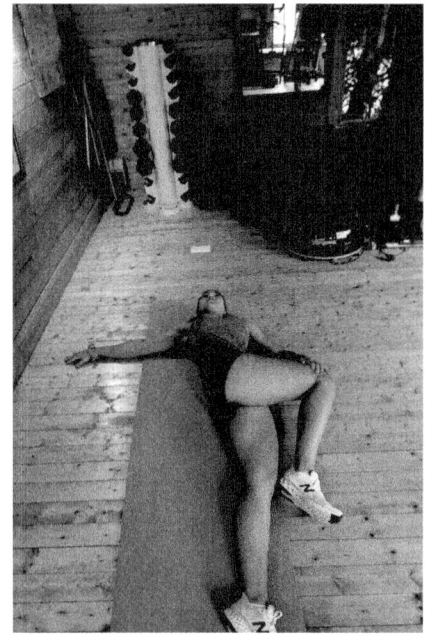

Pointers: You might feel that when you take your leg over to stretch your back you are only feeling the stretch in your gluteal muscle and that because of this the stretch isn't working. Hold the stretch for the recommended period of time and the more you perform this stretch, the more relaxed your glute will be and the greater the rotation in your lumbar back will be.

LEG STRETCHES

Stretching of the leg muscles (glutes, piriformis, hamstring, and hip flexors) is also hugely important in reducing the pull on certain areas of the spine.

Hamstrings: As we discussed earlier, the hamstrings connect to your sit bones and if they are tight, this can lead to a posterior tilt pulling effect on the pelvis (backwards rotation of the pelvis) and therefore lead to a flattened lumbar spine.

Hip Flexors: If the hip flexors are tight (which they generally are in those who sit for long periods) then this can cause the opposite effect and lead to an increased anterior pelvic tilt (Forward rotation of the pelvis).

Piriformis/Gluteal: The piriformis muscles sit on either side underneath the gluteal muscles and both connect to the pelvis. Both the piriformis and gluteus muscles can be stretched in similar ways, so I have grouped them together.

Hamstring Stretches

Easy Level Supine Hamstring Stretch

In case you've forgotten our anatomy lesson earlier on in the book, the hamstring muscle is the big muscle in the back of your thigh. The hamstring quite rightly gets much attention for its annoying habit of becoming tight and causing back problems.

We shouldn't blame the muscle however, but our lack of mobility throughout the day. This is the real culprit when it comes to tightness in the hamstrings. Even if your hamstring isn't particularly tight I will always advocate to keep it stretched out to prevent any tightness from occurring down the line.

1. Start by lying on your back with both knees bent to 90 degrees.
2. Bring one of your knees towards your chest. Interlock your fingers behind your knee.
3. To stretch the hamstring, keep your hands where they are and extend your leg towards the ceiling.
4. You should feel a stretch in the back of your thigh.
5. Hold this stretch for between 30-45 seconds.
6. Return to the starting position and repeat for the other leg.
7. Repeat 1-2 more set for both legs, with breaks in between.

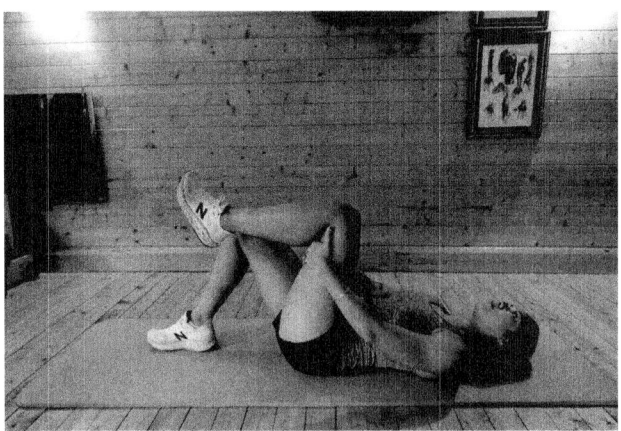

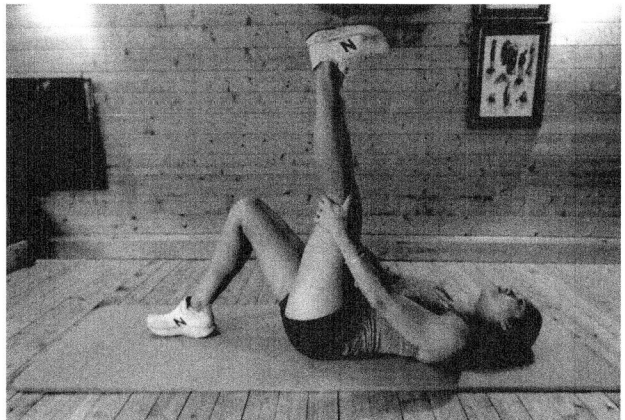

Pointers: When people are stretching the leg muscles I often see them pulsing backwards and forwards. A static stretch should be taken to the point where you feel the stretch and then held there for the said amount of time in that position.

*This can be used for all conditions.

Moderate Level Long Sitting Hamstring Stretch

This next one for the hamstring will provide slightly more tension on the stretch compared to the supine stretch we just went through. If you have a disc bulge this may not be the most appropriate for you due to the significant amount of lumbar flexion sustained through the back.

1. You can either be sitting on the floor or on your bed with your legs straight out in front of you
2. Being one foot in towards your other thigh to act as a base of support.
3. Keeping your other leg straight, run both hands down the straight leg towards your foot.

4. You should feel a strong stretch in the back of your straight leg.
5. Hold this stretch for between 30-45 seconds and then return to the starting position.
6. Repeat for the other leg.
7. Perform 1-2 more sets on both legs with a break in between.

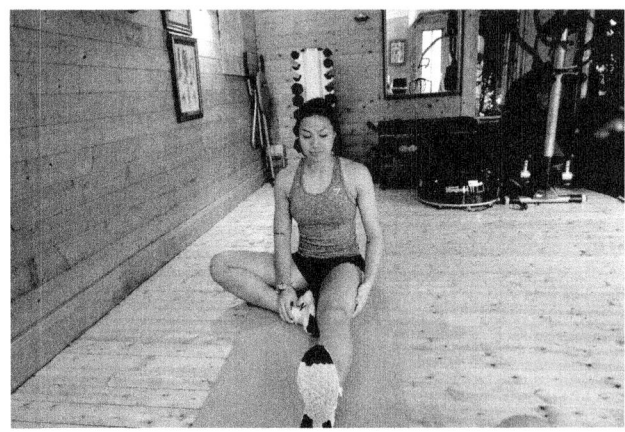

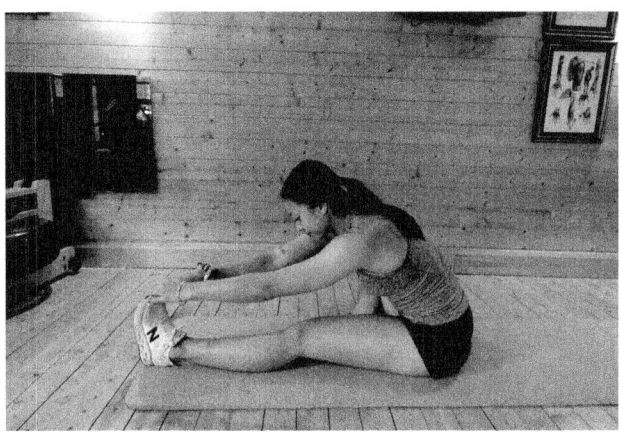

| Moderate level sitting hamstring stretch

Pointers: Bringing your toes towards you on the leg to be stretched can increase the amount of stretch felt in the back of the hamstring. However, if you have any sciatic nerve disruption, I would steer clear of doing this.

Advanced Level Standing Half Clock-Face

This is by far my favorite hamstring stretch as it involves a dynamic (a stretch involving movement) element to it. It might feel a bit strange when you first attempt it, however the great thing about this stretch is you can feel it stretching the different parts of your hamstring.

1. Start in a step-stance position with the leg to be stretched slightly in front of the other. The leg to be stretched should be straight and the leg behind is slightly bent.
2. Look down at your foot on the leg to be stretched and imagine half of a clock-face around your foot, from 9 to 3.
3. Run both hands down the front of your leg and start at the number 9 on the clock-face.
4. Now go until you feel the stretch and then come up slightly and then go to 10, then 11, then 12 until you reach 3. Then reverse and go to all the numbers back to 9. Imagine it almost like you're bobbing up and down from number to number.
5. Repeat going from 9 to 3 and back, 3 times in total.
6. Perform the stretch on both legs, 3 times each leg with a break in between.

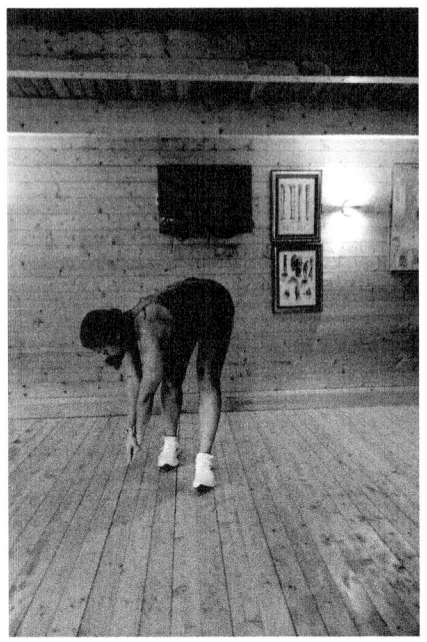

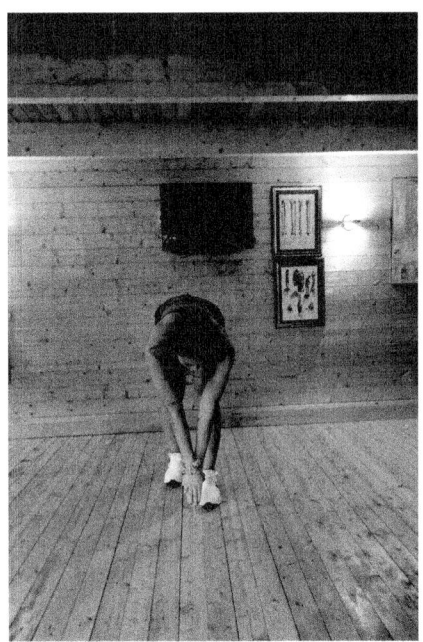

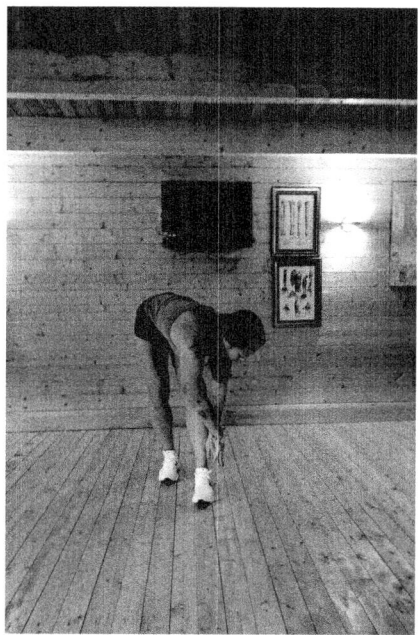

Pointers: If you're having trouble feeling the stretch, you can try slightly bending the knee of the front leg as well. This will still provide a stretch to the hamstring but you will feel it slightly higher up the leg towards your bottom. *Try not to bend from your back—push your hips backwards using the hip hinge motion, and keep your spine as straight as possible.

Piriformis/Gluteal Stretches

Easy Level Supine Piriformis/Glute Stretch

The piriformis and glutes perform very different roles in your pelvis. You have one of the biggest muscles in your body, in the glutes and one of the smallest with the piriformis. However, when it comes to stretching them, they are stretched in much the same way and if either are too tight, they can contribute to lower back pain as well as host of other lower leg musculoskeletal problems.

1. Start by sitting at the edge of the chair, with your feet hip-width apart.
2. Cross one leg over the other, resting your ankle on top of the other knee.
3. You may feel a stretch already in that position if you're particularly tight in these muscles.
4. To increase the stretch, take your hand and press on your knee, pushing down and away from you.
5. You should feel a stretch in your buttock region.
6. Hold for between 30-45 seconds.
7. Repeat on both sides. Perform 3 sets on both sides with a break in between.

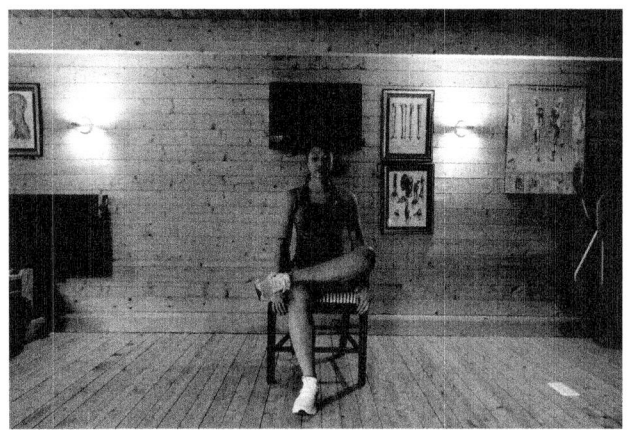

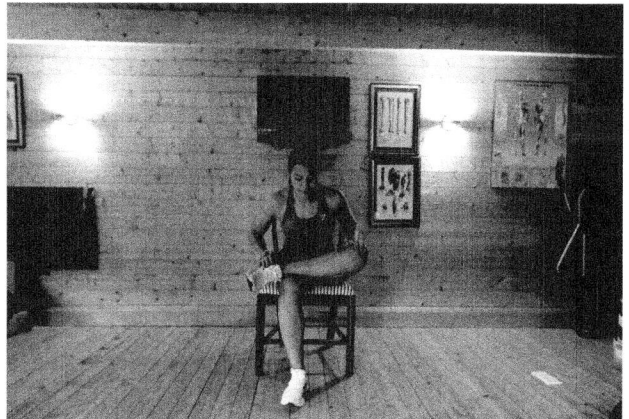

Pointers: To increase the stretch of this exercise you can lean forward after you've pushed the knee down and this will increase the stretch in your bottom area.

*This can be used for all conditions.

Moderate Level Piriformis/Glute Stretch

This exercise is similar to the "easy" one we just went through but has an increased stretch on the muscles. This might be familiar to a lot of you who have done rehab exercises before but it was an exercise which I had to include, thanks to how useful it can be.

1. Start by lying on your back with your knees bent to 90 degrees.
2. Again cross one leg over the other, resting your ankle on top of the stationary knee.
3. Place one hand through the gap made by crossing your leg and the other hand around the thigh of the stationary leg and interlock your hands.
4. To perform the stretch, pull your leg towards you. You should feel a strong stretch in your buttock muscles.

5. Hold for between 30-45 seconds.
6. Repeat 3 sets on both sides with a 30 second break in between each set.

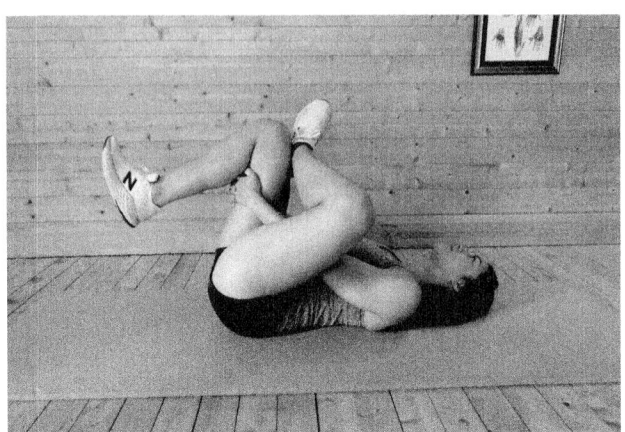

Pointers: Those of you suffering with a disc bulge, this exercise might increase your pain. If it does then I would suggest sticking to the seated stretch.

Advanced Modified Pigeon Stretch:

This is not one for you if you have painful knees, but if you are able to manage it, it can provide a significant stretch of the gluteal and piriformis muscles. It also has the added benefit of providing a lovely lumbar flexion stretch at the same time.

1. Start in the All 4's position on the floor.
2. Place one leg out straight behind you, and the leg to be stretched, rotate and bring it under your body.
3. You should already feel a stretch in your buttock muscles.
4. To increase the stretch, drop your hip towards the

floor and bring your body closer to the ground. This will really increase the stretch of the gluteal and piriformis muscle.

5. Hold for 20-30 seconds.
6. Repeat on both sides, twice over

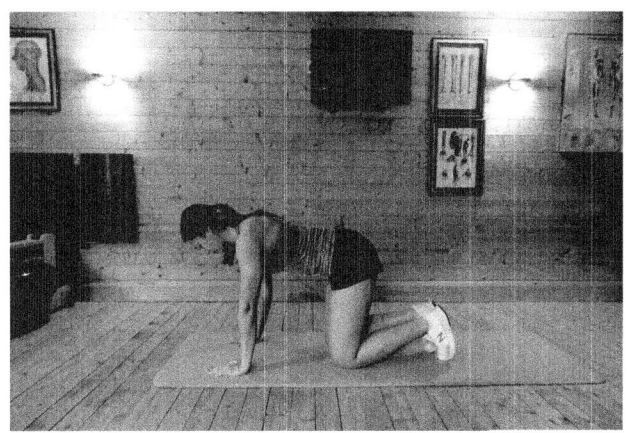

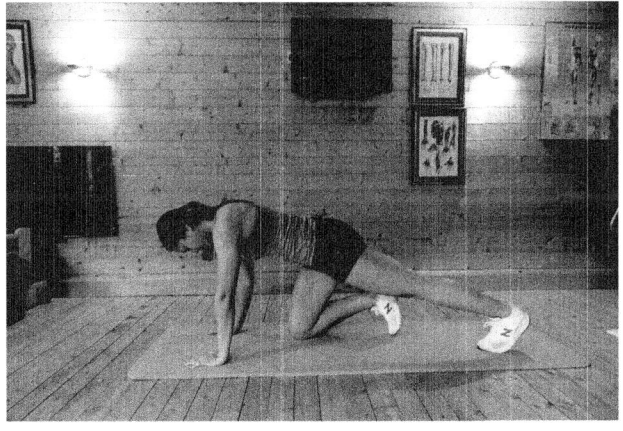

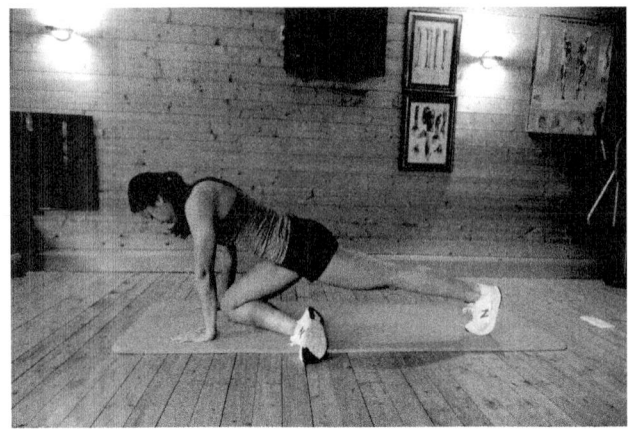

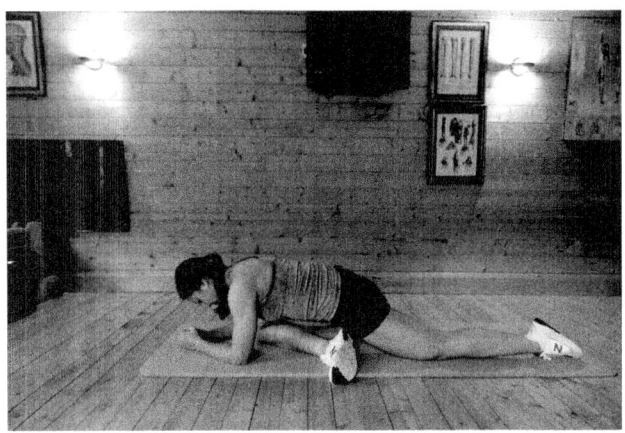

Pointers: You have to be fairly mobile and have good knees to perform this exercise. If you find it an awkward position to get into or painful at all then just stick to the previous exercise.

Hip Flexor Stretches

Easy Level Leg-Hang Off Bed

The last muscles we are working on are the hip flexor muscles. As the name would suggest they flex the hip. When we sit all day, they are in a shortened position for long periods, making them prone to becoming very tight. They are a touch difficult to stretch fully if you're not the most mobile, but hopefully one of the levels of this stretch will be manageable for you.

1. The starting position is lying on the edge of your bed.
2. The leg to be stretched is the one nearest the edge of the bed. The other leg should be bent to 90 degrees to support your back.
3. Slowly lower the leg off of the bed until you can feel a stretch in the muscles at the front of your thigh.
4. Hold this stretch for 30-45 seconds.
5. Repeat on both sides, 1-2 more times, with a 30 second break in between.

*This can be used for all conditions.

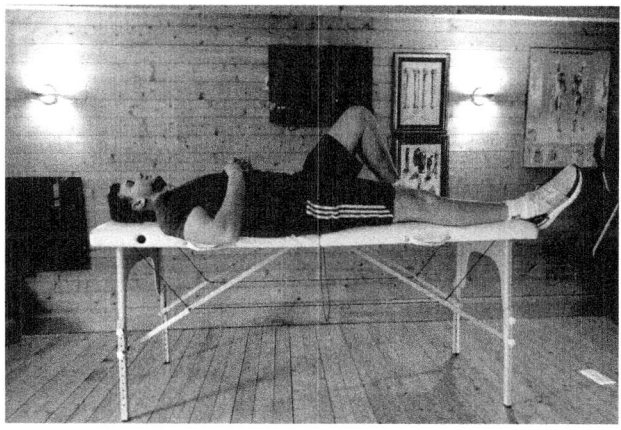

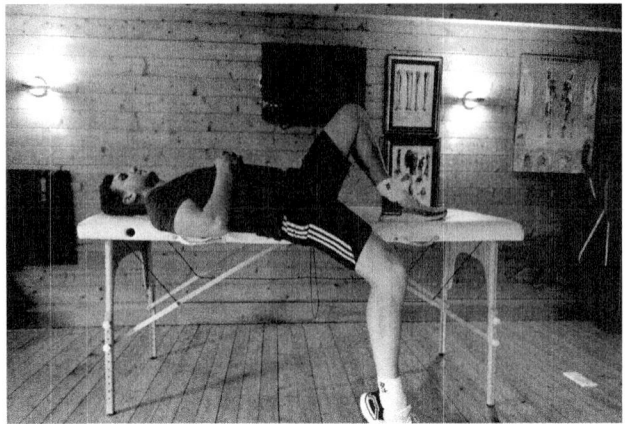

Pointers: This exercise works best if the foot of the leg hanging off the bed is just slightly in contact with the ground. Those of you with high beds or shorter legs can certainly try it and see how it feels, or place a pillow or a small box below where your foot reaches to heighten the level of the floor.

Moderate Level Standing Hip Flexor Stretch

The moderate level standing hip flexor stretch gives a more significant stretch than the leg-hang stretch, but is easier to implement than the full kneeling stretch.

1. Start by standing with your feet roughly shoulder width apart.
2. Bring one leg forward and bend you knee as if you're going to enter a lunge position, but keep your back leg straight. You should feel the stretch in the hip flexor of the straight back leg.
3. Hold the stretch for 20-30 seconds.
4. Repeat 3 times on each side, with a 30-45 second break in between.

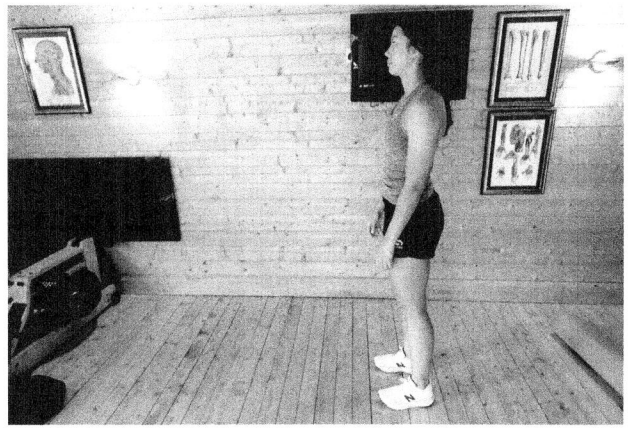

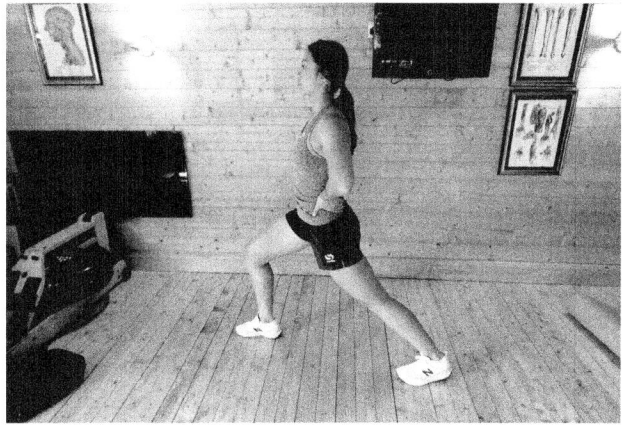

| Moderate level hip flexor stretch

Advanced Level Kneeling Stretch

This is the best exercise for feeling the greatest amount of stretch in your hip flexors. Again, sorry for those of you who have painful knees, this might not be the best option for you.

1. Start in the kneeling position on the floor.
2. Take one leg forward so you are in a kneeling lunge position.
3. Lean forwards trying to lead with the front of your

hip. You should feel a strong stretch at the front of your hip.

4. To increase the stretch further, reach up as high as you can to the ceiling.
5. Hold the stretch for between 30-45 seconds.
6. Repeat on both sides, twice over.

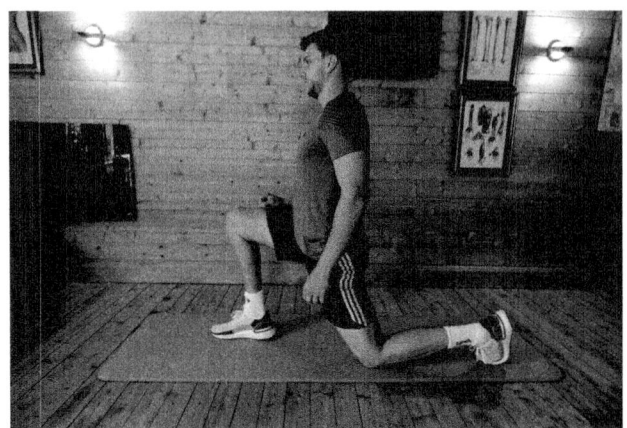

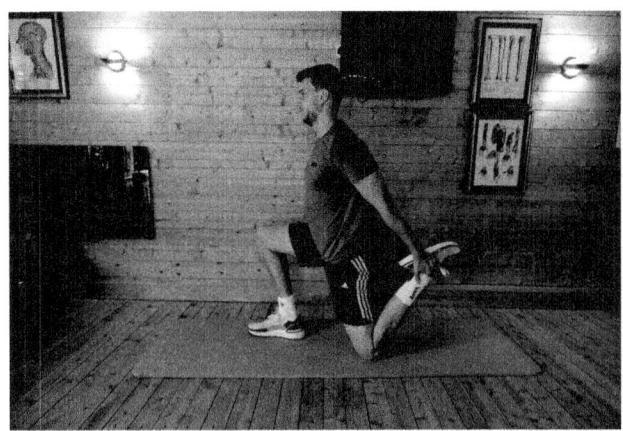

Pointers: To increase the stretch further you can place your foot on a box, other low surface or reach back and hold it with your hand, as shown here. This will greatly increase the stretch, however not many will be able to do this, so don't worry if this feels too difficult.

THORACIC SPINE POSTURE-SPECIFIC STRETCHES

In Chapter 3 we discussed the kyphotic posture which is attributed to a stiff thoracic spine and weak back muscles. Below are the exercises for both problems. .

There are 3 stretching suggestions of the thoracic spine, to be performed if you feel as though your posture is not "ideal." In Chapter 5 the back strengthening exercises will be discussed. Most people can benefit from some increased thoracic spine mobility, especially over 50's, as this is when the thoracic stiffness usually starts to increase.

*In the exercise program table, these stretches are labeled as the *posture* exercises which you can choose to implement if you feel necessary. I generally have my patients perform these stretches regardless, as long as they are not causing any pain.

Kneeling Thoracic Spine Extension Stretch

1. Kneel facing a chair. Place a cushion under your knees if you need to.
2. Place your hands behind your head and have your elbows rested on the chair in front of you.
3. To stretch the thoracic spine, drop your chest towards the ground. This will cause your thoracic spine to stretch into extension.
4. Hold for 20-30seconds, then relax.
5. Aim for 3 repetitions of this exercise.

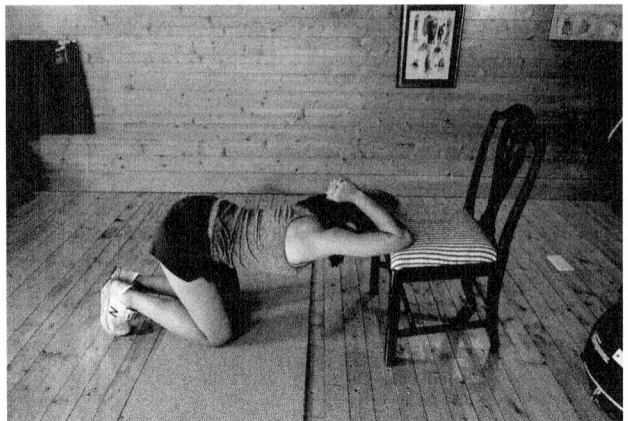

| Kneeling thoracic spine extension stretch

Standing Thoracic Spine Extension Stretch

For those unable to kneel, try this thoracic spine stretch. This stretch is not as significant as the kneeling stretch, but is a great option if you can't kneel.

1. Place your hands behind your head and go up against a wall with your elbows resting on the wall.
2. To perform the stretch, drop your chest towards the wall, you should feel a nice stretch in the middle of your back.
3. Hold for 20-30 seconds, then relax.
4. Aim for 3 repetitions of this exercise.

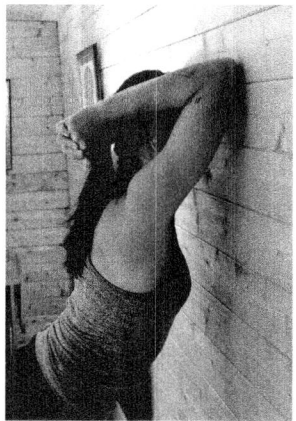

Standing thoracic extension stretch on wall

Lying Thoracic Spine Extension With Towel

1. Start by lying on your back.
2. Roll up a towel and place under your thoracic spine in between your shoulder blades.
3. Lie and hold for a couple of minutes at a time. Rest and then repeat for another 2 minutes again
4. Aim to do this 2-3 times per week

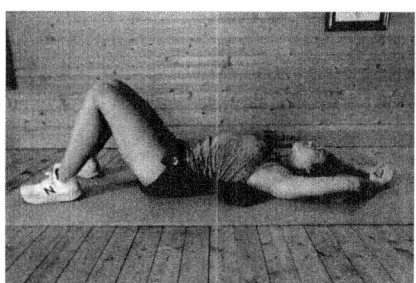

That brings us to the end of the stretches! Remember, as always, don't do any of the stretches if they increase your pain. Pick the ones you are comfortable with, and do them consistently.

5

Step 5: Strengthening

I KNOW that up until this point, all the steps I've mentioned were "important," and strengthening is no exception. To be honest, they are *all* important steps. Strengthening can have a huge impact on relieving pain from our backs. When our muscles are strong, the pressure put on all of our bones, joints, ligaments, and tendons in our back is lessened. In particular, our core and our legs are important when it comes to our backs, so these are the muscle groups we will be focusing on throughout this chapter. There will be different levels and professions for these exercises, so as always, do what you feel you can, and take it easy—you don't want to push too hard and make your back worse. Here we go! We'll start with the easy core exercise program.

EASY CORE HOME EXERCISES

You're going to want to grab a chair for these exercises. Preferably one that doesn't have any arm rests, as they might get in the way.

. . .

Back Twists (Warm Up)

1. Sit upright so that your back is not resting on the chair, and make sure you are centered and not leaning in any direction.
2. Rotate your torso in both directions, making sure you're really working on your posture and getting warmed up. Repeat rotations 5-10 times.

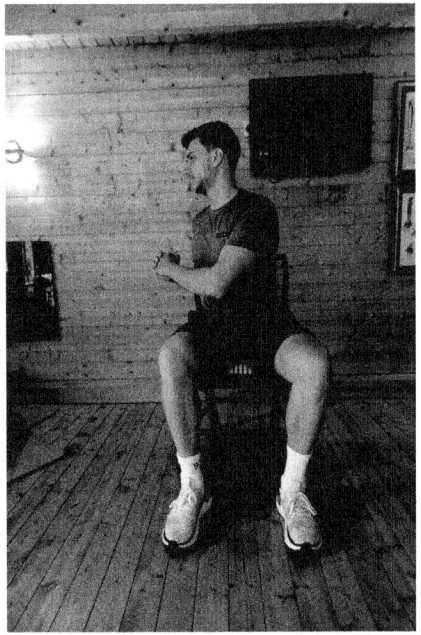

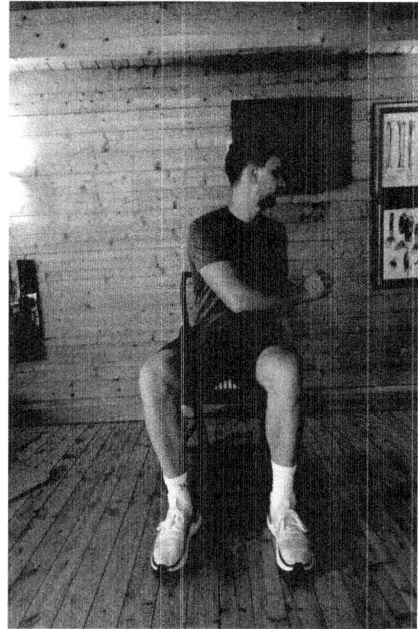

Warm up for easy ab workout. Rotations from left to right in sitting.

Forward Bends In Sitting (Warm Up)

1. Sit in your chair with your legs extended slightly out in front.
2. Take the palms of your hands and place them on your thighs. Now run your palms down your thighs all the way down to your shins, as far as you can go without causing any pain. You should feel a slight stretch in your hamstrings as well–this is okay.
3. Now reverse, and slide your palms up your shins and back onto your thighs. When you get to the top, roll your shoulders back before starting again. Perform this 3-4 times.

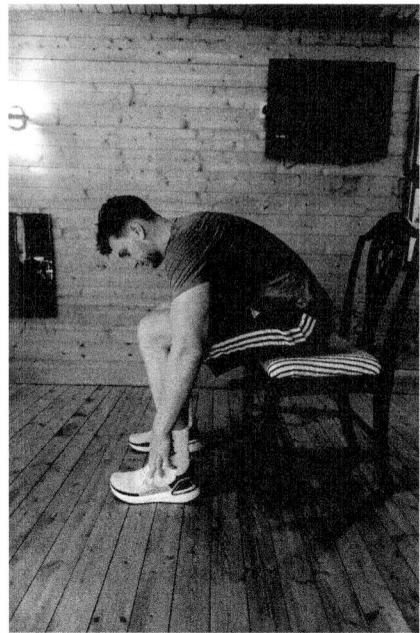

| Warm up for easy ab workout, forward bends

Chair Sit-ups

1. Still sitting in the chair, slide your bottom to the front edge of the seat, making sure not to slide all the way off. Hold on to the sides of the chair for stability if you feel like you need it.
2. Keeping your spine straight, lean back in the chair. You should feel your abdominal muscles tightening up.
3. Come back up to an upright position, keeping your back straight, and engaging your core. Repeat this motion 5-10 times, or more if you feel you can.

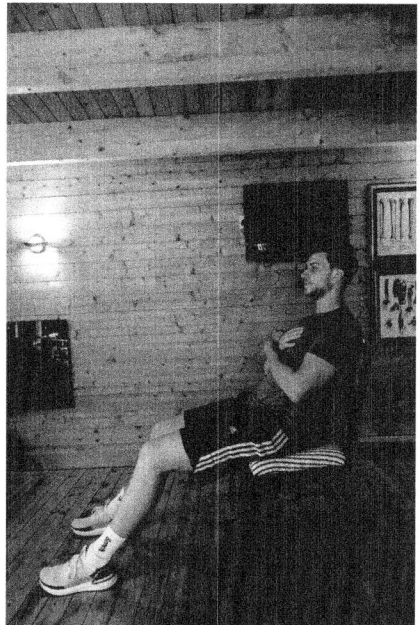

| Sit ups in chair starting position

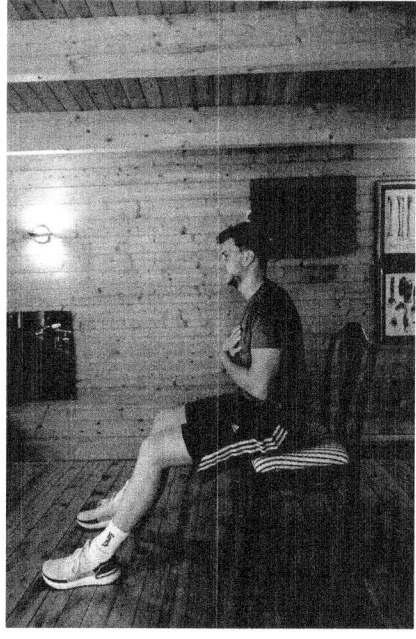

| Sit ups in chair finishing position.

Tummy Squeezes

1. Sitting upright in your chair, place your hands on your knees. Keep your posture nice and tall.
2. Engage your core by simply squeezing and tensing your abdominal muscles. Hold this for 5-10 seconds, and repeat 3-4 times.

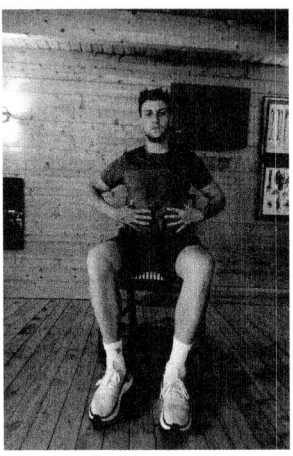

Squeeze your tummy muscles by drawing your tummy button in toward your spine

Leg Kick Out in Front

1. While seated, slide to the edge of the chair again. Keep your spine straight, and lean back slightly.
2. Extend your legs straight out in front of you, resting your heels on the ground. Hold on to the sides of the seat again for more stability.
3. Raise one leg up off the ground, about 6-8 inches up, or whatever feels comfortable to you, but you want to lift your foot slightly into the air. You should feel the

lower part of your abdominals engaging to keep your leg raised.

4. Lower your leg back down.
5. Repeat step 3 with your other leg. Continue to alternate lifting your legs into the air, one leg at a time.
6. Perform 5-10 reps on each leg, and perform 2-3 sets.

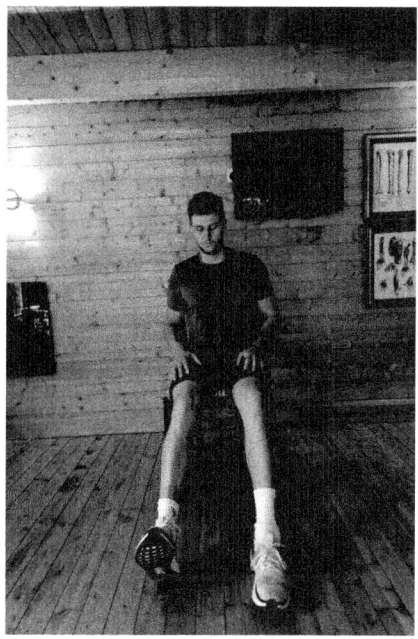

Seated leg lifts with leg straight. Keep your core engaged throughout this exercise

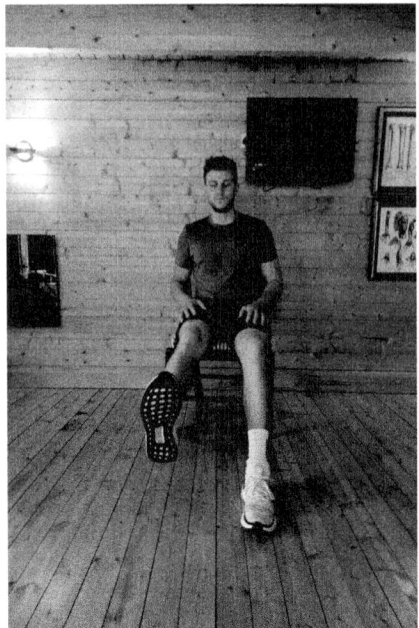

| Seated leg lift finishing position.

Note: If necessary, you can keep your legs bent at roughly a 90 degree angle instead of extending them out in front of you, and lift at the knee instead of your feet. This will be slightly easier than with your legs extended outward.

Seated Ab Bicycle

1. Slide slightly forward in the chair so you have a little bit of room to lean backwards, but don't go too far forward.
2. Once you are slightly leaning back, lift both of your knees several inches off the ground, and start performing bike pedaling motions with your feet. These don't need to be large circles, but it should be a continuous movement between both legs.

3. Don't forget to keep your back straight, and slightly lean backwards for this exercise, making sure you can feel the engagement in your abdomen.

4. Perform 5-10 alternating pedaling motions on each leg.

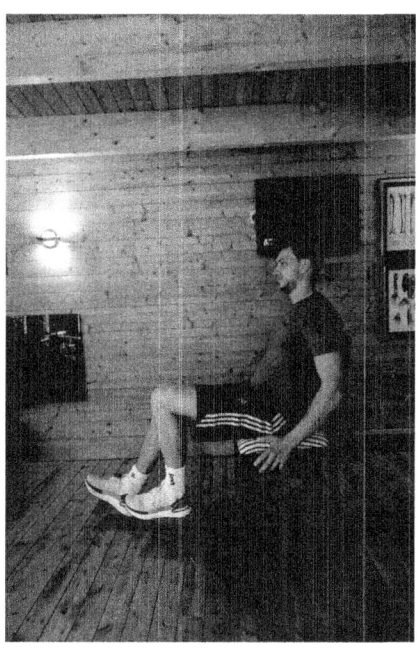

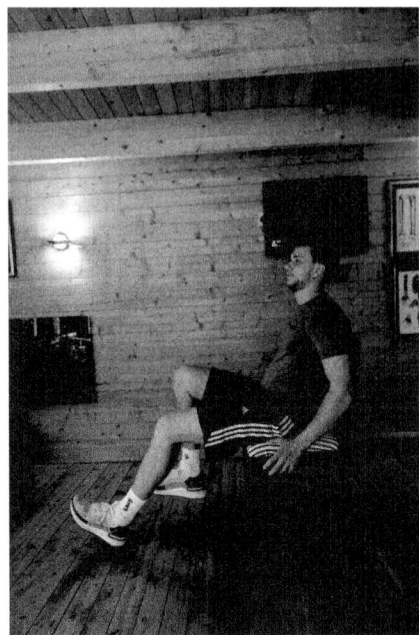

Seated cycling. Try and keep both feet off the floor when doing the exercise. If you do need to touch your feet down to the floor that is fine to do.

Seated Obliques

1. Sit straight up, and hold your hands together out in front of you.
2. With your knees shoulder-width apart, place your hands between the knees.
3. Rotate your torso to one side until your hands touch your knee, and push into the knee with your hands, creating resistance with your knee. You should feel tension in the oblique muscles on the same side you rotate to. So if you rotated left, you should feel the engagement in your left obliques.

4. Hold this position for 5 seconds, keeping your core engaged the whole time.
5. Release your hands back to the middle.
6. Repeat this motion in the other direction, and hold again for 5 seconds.
7. Repeat this exercise 3-5 times on each side. Don't forget to keep your back straight.

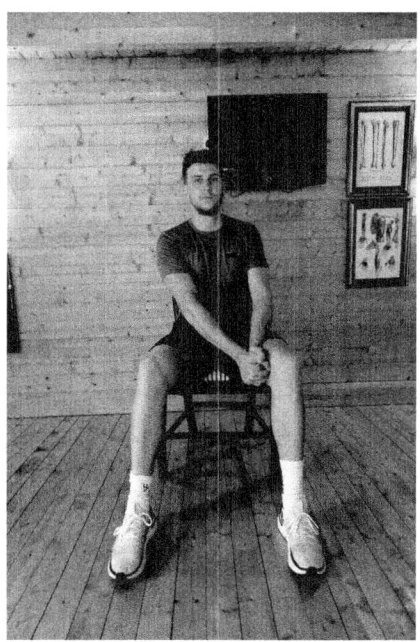

| Seated oblique, left sided hold

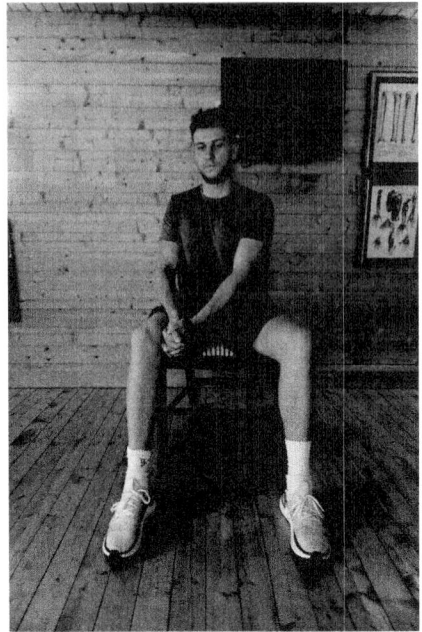

Seated oblique, right sided hold

*For all conditions, if you find that any of the exercises aggravate your back, leave those ones out.

ADVANCED CORE HOME EXERCISES

If you are wanting to challenge yourself further, then next up is the advanced core exercise program. The following 4 exercises are ones I have been using with my patients for a few years now. I started using them after reading the research conducted by Dr. Stuart McGill, who found these to be the most optimal exercises for strengthening your core while exhibiting the least amount of stress on the spine. That is why for my programs I don't include the standard plank or leg raises which are popular among core workout plans—while they are good at working the abdominal muscles, they also place increased stress on the spine during the movement.

The core as a whole is optimal when you have the front core muscles (transversus and rectus abdominis), the side core muscles (the obliques) and the back muscles (the erector spinae) all strong and working together. We'll start with exercises for the front core.

EXERCISES FOR THE FRONT CORE MUSCLES

The Abdominal Crunch

1. Lie on your back with your knees bent to 90 degrees and your feet on the floor.
2. Place your hand under your lower back to maintain the arch (as pictured). You want to maintain the arch when performing the exercise. This is often where people go wrong with the sit up, as it simply aggravates their back pain. If you have a painful shoulder, roll up a towel and place it under your back instead.
3. To perform the sit-up, lift your shoulders roughly a

couple inches off the floor. (Don't lead with your head.

4. You should feel your abdominals strongly contract.

5. Hold for between 5-10 seconds at the top of the movement, then slowly return to the starting position.

6. Repeat up to 5 times or until you get fatigued with at least a 5 second break in between each set.

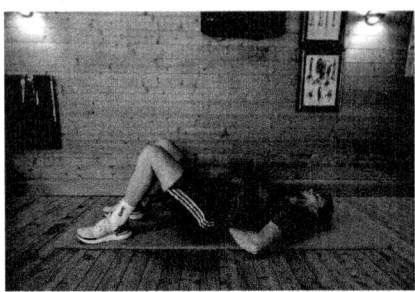

Sit up with hand under back starting position.
Remember if you have painful shoulders you can roll
up a towel and place under your back

Pointers: If you find your neck hurts when performing this exercise, stop leading with your chin. Focus on lifting your shoulders off the floor and you will feel your abdominals contract much more strongly and your neck will stop hurting.

*For all conditions. There should be very minimal lumbar flexion occurring when doing these exercises. Your shoulders should only just be coming off the ground, hence why it is an appropriate exercise for all. As always though, if it doesn't agree with your back then stop.

The Deadbug

1. Lie on your back with your arms straight in the air and your hips bent to 90 degrees, as shown (Figure 1).

2. Engage your core muscles by gently pulling your belly button towards your spine, maintaining your breathing.

3. Place a thin rolled up towel under your lower back just to maintain the arch.

4. Lower your right leg towards the floor while simultaneously taking your left arm behind you backwards towards the floor (Figure 2).

5. Keep your core engaged the whole time, once both your arm and leg are a couple inches from the floor, slowly return them both to the starting position.

6. Then repeat for the opposite arm and leg.

7. Repeat up to 5 alternate repetitions for both sides.

Pointers: The deadbug not only challenges the core, but also your coordination. If you're finding it challenging to do the opposite arm and leg at the same time, you can just simply do one limb at a time. This will still work your core muscles but will be easier on your coordination skills (Figure 3).

To further make this an easier exercise you can have your legs bent and tap your feet to the ground with a bent leg (Figures 4 and 5).

*There's not any specific condition that this exercise shouldn't be used for. However, when you take your opposite arm and opposite leg in different directions this could potentially create tension for some backs. I have included it because it's such a great core exercise. If you do find arm and leg together too difficult, stick to just taking 1 limb away from the body at once.

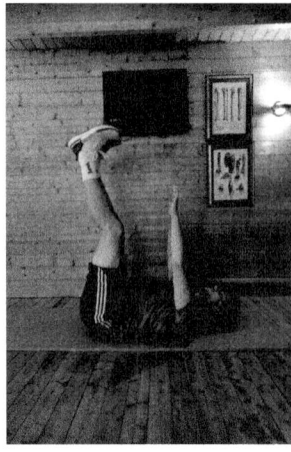

Figure 1: Deadbug starting position. Both arms and legs straight

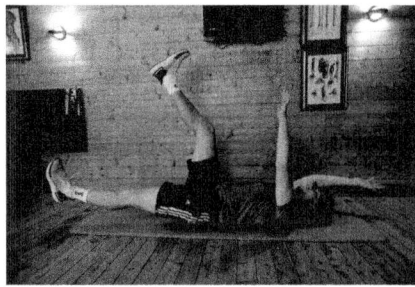

Figure 2: Deadbug ending position with opposite arm and leg extended.

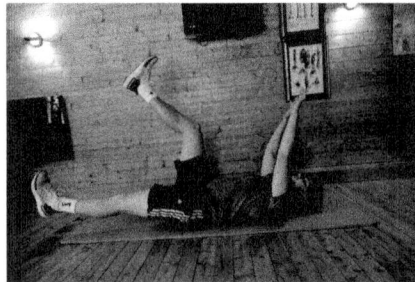

Figure 3: Deadbug one limb movement at a time.

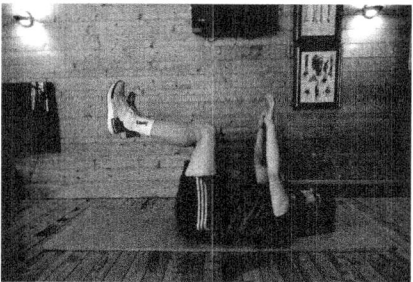

Figure 4: Deadbug easier starting position with knees bent to 90 degrees.

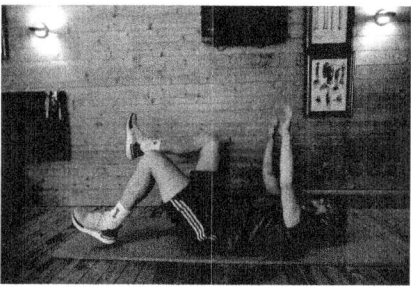

Figure 5: Deadbug easier finishing position with heel tap to the floor.

FOR THE SIDE CORE MUSCLES

Side Plank

Shoulder affected version:

1. Stand parallel with the wall.
2. Take 1 step out away from the wall and place your forearm against the wall as shown in the picture below.
3. To get your obliques to contract you need to lean into the wall with your forearm and this should cause your side abdominal muscles to contract, while holding your body straight.
4. Hold for 10 seconds and then relax. Have at least a 5 second break and then repeat 5 times on both sides

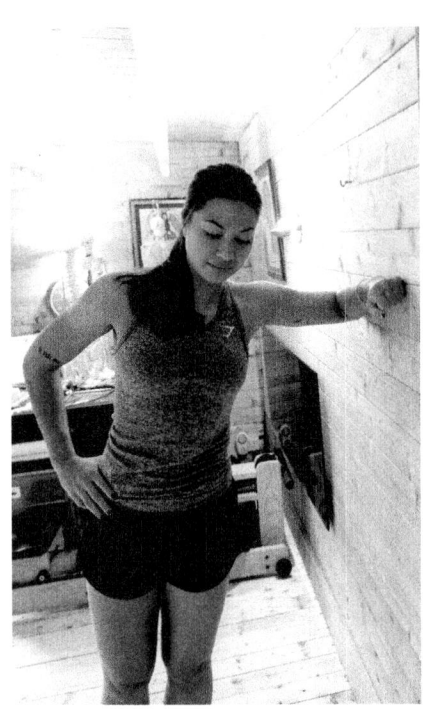

Pointers: Make a mental note not to allow your bottom to sag when performing the exercise, try and keep your back as straight as possible as shown in here.

More Challenging Side Plank Exercise

1. Lie on your side with your knees bent.
2. Get into the starting position with your elbow and forearm propping your body up at an angle, as shown in the picture below.
3. To initiate the exercise, raise your hip up from the floor so your body becomes a diagonal line.
4. You should feel your side abdominal muscles contracting while doing this.
5. Hold for 10 seconds and then return to the starting position.
6. Repeat up to 5 times on each side or until you become fatigued and have at least a 5 second break in between each set.

*Applicable for all patients so long as they can do either variation.

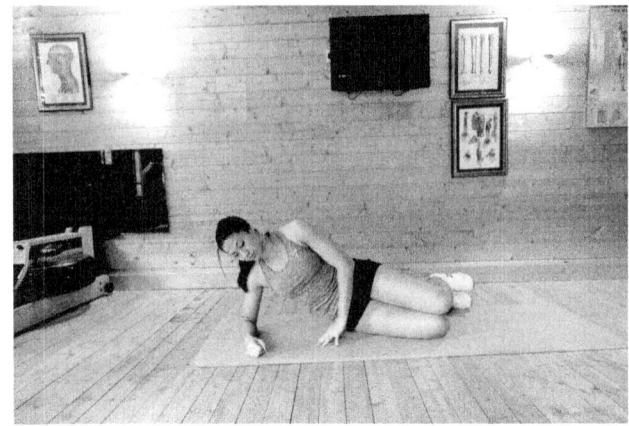

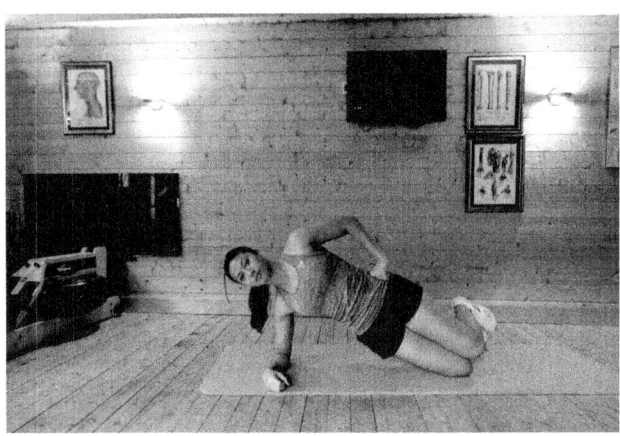

FOR THE BACK CORE MUSCLES

The Bird Dog

1. Start on all 4's (hands and knees on the ground). You can place a towel or cushion under your knees for comfort if needed.
2. Get your back into the neutral spine position and gently tighten your core muscles.

3. Take one arm out in front of you, while maintaining the tightened core and level spine.

4. Then return to neutral and take the opposite leg behind you. Imagine you are slowly donkey kicking something behind you.

5. The goal is to simultaneously bring your right arm out in front of you and push your left leg out behind you while maintaining a strong core and neutral back.

6. Once you are able to, try bringing your opposite arm and opposite leg together, repeat on the other side.

7. The emphasis for this exercise is to perform smooth controlled movements with a stable spine, not to do it as quickly as possible.

8. Hold for a maximum of 10 seconds and repeat up to 3 times on both sides, alternating as you go.

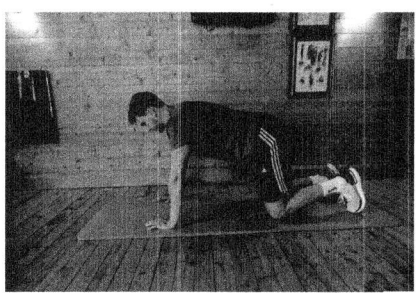

Starting position of the Bird Dog exercise. Note the neutral spine.

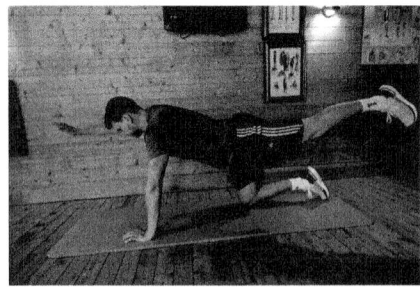

Finished Bird Dog exercise with both opposite arm and leg extended.

Pointers: Many people believe they are doing this exercise correctly, when in fact, they are over arching their lumbar spine in an attempt to reach as far forward as possible. The main focus should be on keeping the spine in a neutral position and keeping the core tight, and less so about how far you can reach forward.

*Applicable for all patients regardless of condition. You might need to play around with the different variations and build up until you can do the opposite arm and opposite leg.

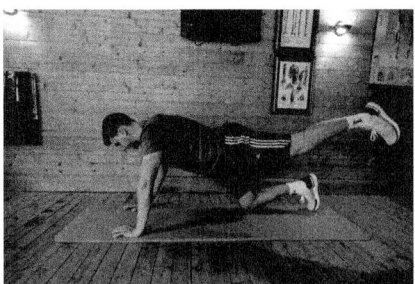

Bird Dog variation with single leg extension

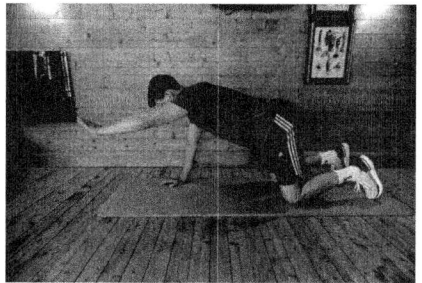

| Bird Dog variation with arm extension only

LEG STRENGTHENING

"A healthy back needs a healthy core"–most if not all medical professionals would agree with this statement. The abdominal muscles are referred to as the core. However, I would strongly argue that for a healthy back you need as much of a strong *foundation* as you need a strong core. I refer to the leg muscles as the foundation in this case. Even if you have a strong and functioning core that's keeping everything in check in your midriff section, your back is not going to be happy if your legs are weak and not providing a solid base of support. I often see this in clinics with patients who have strengthened their core, done the flexibility work, and are generally keeping fit. But when I go to test their lower limb muscle strength and observe them performing functional tasks, this is where the weakness lies. A short program of leg strengthening fills in the missing piece to the puzzle, and can make a big difference. This is why for my program, the leg strengthening component is trained as much as the core exercises–to set a solid foundation.

I have devised an easy program and an advanced program for home exercises, as well as a gym program for those of you who have access to a gym. For your leg strengthening days, perform one of the three programs that follow. They have an even spread of exercises targeting different muscle groups. If there is an exercise which you can't do for whatever reason, don't worry. If there is an exercise which you have done for at least a couple of days and you feel it is making your back worse, don't do it. The last thing you want is to make matters worse!

Some important terms regarding strength training to avoid any confusion:

- **Reps**: For each exercise perform the number of repetitions (Reps) suggested. 1 'set' is equivalent to how many repetitions have been stated.
- **Sets**: If it says perform '3 sets' then you need to perform however many repetitions are stated (e.g. 10) and repeat those 10 repetitions (10 reps), 3 times through (3 sets).
- **Break**: It's important to have a break in between each set to allow the muscles to appropriately recover so they don't fatigue too quickly, or injure. The break time between all sets is 30-45 seconds.
- **Too easy**? If you get to the 10th repetition and you feel as though it was too easy or like you could have done more, then increase the resistance. You can use a more challenging resistance band. If you are unable to get ahold of resistance bands or light weights, then you can increase the reps until you feel your muscles fatiguing. There's not an exact science to this but 10 reps is usually a good number to aim for.

Resistance Bands

If you haven't seen or heard of a resistance band before, it's just an elastic band which can be used for exercises, sometimes referred to as a theraband. It provides a resistance to the movement you are performing, making it more challenging, and thus making the muscle work harder. There are different strengths of resistance bands so you can choose to make it easier or harder depending on what your needs are. There are many different brands which all have their own color coding system for the different strengths of the bands. You can purchase either a close-looped band or a long unattached band. For the exercises in this book, the closed loop band would be preferable, however, if you do have a long band then you can simply tie a knot in the band and it will perform the same role.

Ankle Weights

These can also be used to make a particular exercise more challenging by adding a weight to the movement involved. They are strapped around the ankle and come in different weights depending on your needs. I generally prefer using a resistance band to progress exercises as they provide a more consistent resistance throughout the entire range of movement but using an ankle weight is a good option.

*All leg strengthening exercises are recommended for all conditions. However, do take care with the exercises and try to get the form correct, and if any of them do hurt then be sure to stop that particular exercise (try the exercise for at least a few days to 1 week before stopping, sometimes there can be a short term increase in pain while the body adjusts).

Easy At-Home Leg Exercises

The first set of exercises we will go through now, are the easy level leg exercises that can be done at home. Here we go!

Sit to Stand From Chair

This is a simple exercise which engages the gluteal, quadriceps (front of thigh muscles) and hamstring muscles.

1. Start by sitting on a chair with a firm surface (not your sofa).
2. Have your feet hip width apart with your feet firmly flat on the floor.
3. Engage your core muscles by gently pulling in your tummy towards your spine, make sure you maintain your breathing throughout.
4. Cross your arms across your chest and stand up from the chair, squeezing your bottom muscles and driving through with your hips.
5. To return to the chair, perform a hip hinge by pushing your bottom back and lowering back down to the chair while keeping your spine in a neutral position.
6. Perform 3 sets of 10 reps with a 30-45 second break in between each set.

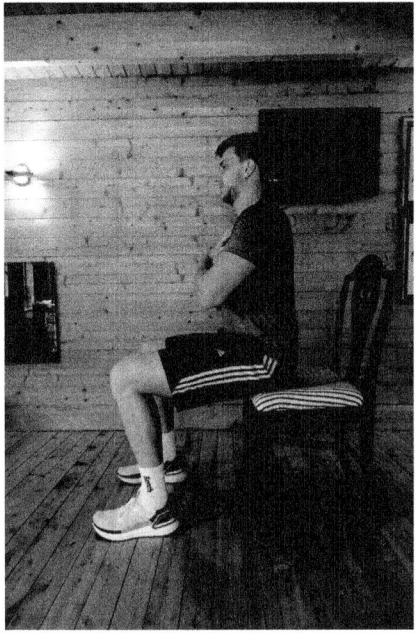

Sit to stand (STS) starting position with hands crossed across chest

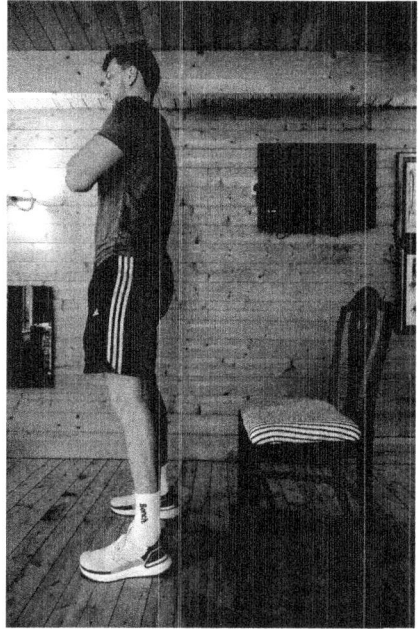

STS finishing position. Remember to drive through from your hips and squeeze your glutes

Resistance Band Progression: Loop the band around your knees and perform the same exercise. The band will provide a resistance inwards towards the knees which will cause your gluteal muscles to work harder.

Pointers: If you find this exercise too difficult, place a few pillows under your bottom so you are performing the exercise from a higher surface, this will make it easier to perform. As you get stronger you should be able to do the exercise from a lower surface and this will demonstrate progress.

The Bridge

A great exercise to work your core, gluteal and hamstring muscles.

1. Start by lying on your back with your knees bent to 90 degrees and your arms resting by your side.
2. Engage your core by pulling in your belly button towards your spine and tightening your abdominal muscles.
3. To initiate the movement, squeeze your gluteal muscles and lift your bottom off the floor, so your body is angled diagonally. Make sure you don't overextend your spine—if you keep your glutes squeezed tightly this shouldn't happen.
4. Hold the position at the top for 10 seconds and then slowly lower your bottom back down to the ground. Relax for 5 seconds. Then repeat 5 repetitions.
5. Aim for 3 sets with a break in between each set.

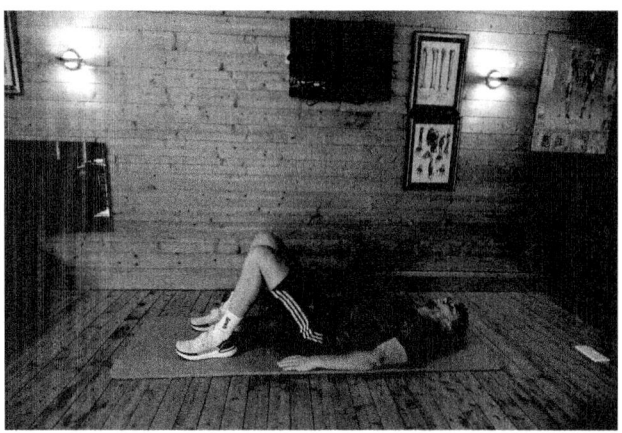

Bridge starting position. Arms out by your side for a good support

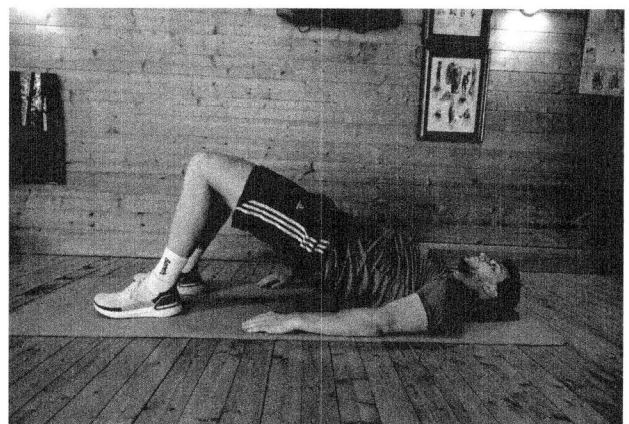

Bridge finishing position. Squeeze your glutes throughout the movement.

Resistance Band Progression: Again, you can place the band above your knees and this will have the same effect of making the glute muscles have to engage more.

Pointers: The focus of this exercise is to work the glutes, hamstrings and core muscles and not about over-arching the back which is often seen. Squeeze the glutes and hamstrings as you're lifting your bottom off while keeping your core tight and simply focus on this.

Straight Leg Raise

The quadriceps muscle (front of thigh), the hip flexor muscles as well as your core all get worked out with this exercise.

Instructions:

1. Lie on the floor on your back with one leg bent and the other leg straight (the straight leg is to be the one that's being worked).
2. Engage your core and tighten your thigh muscles by pushing the back of your knee down into the floor.

3. Raise the leg approximately 6 inches off the floor, and hold for 10-20 seconds.
4. Lower your leg back down to the starting position.
5. Aim to complete 3 sets of 10 repetitions with a 30-45 second break in between.

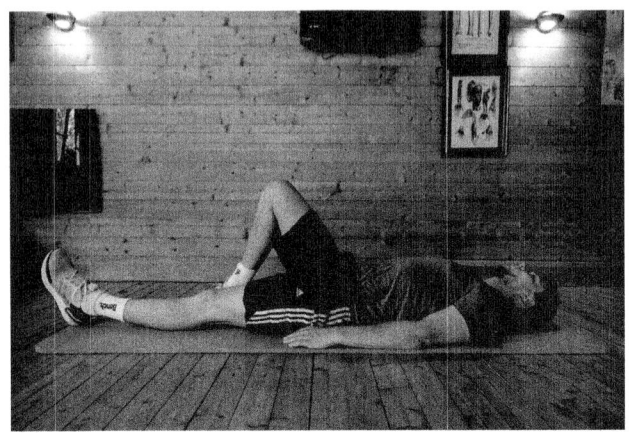

Straight Leg Raise (SLR) exercise starting position. One leg bent to take pressure off your back.

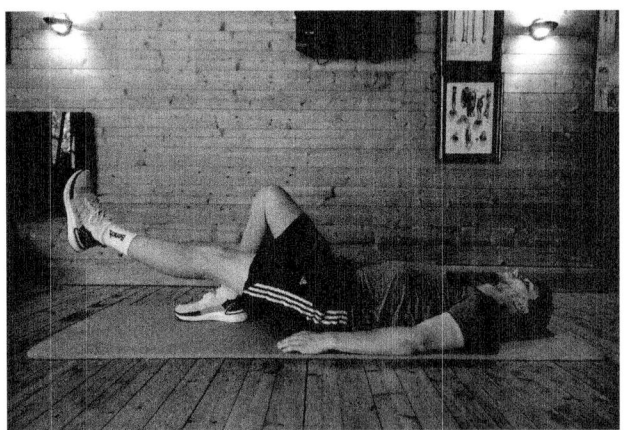

SLR finished position. Raise leg off of floor and hold.

Theraband Progression: Loop the band around your ankles. For this variation, your legs will both be straight and lying on the ground. One leg will remain in contact with the ground in order provide resistance in the band. Your other leg will raise up off the ground in the same way as mentioned above. Your back won't have as much protection as you won't be able to have one leg bent when performing this exercise, but it is a great progression for your thigh muscles if your back can tolerate it.

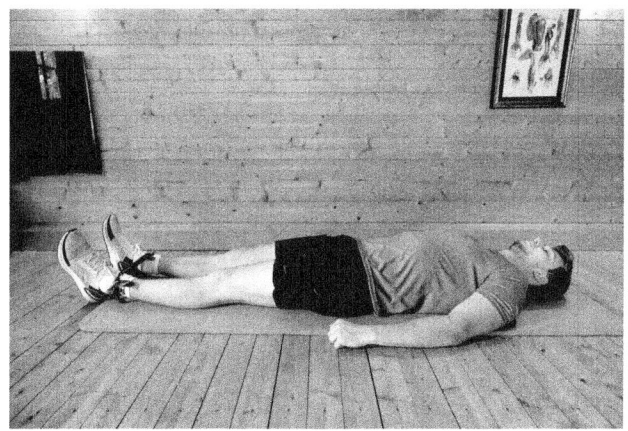

Theraband progression starting position

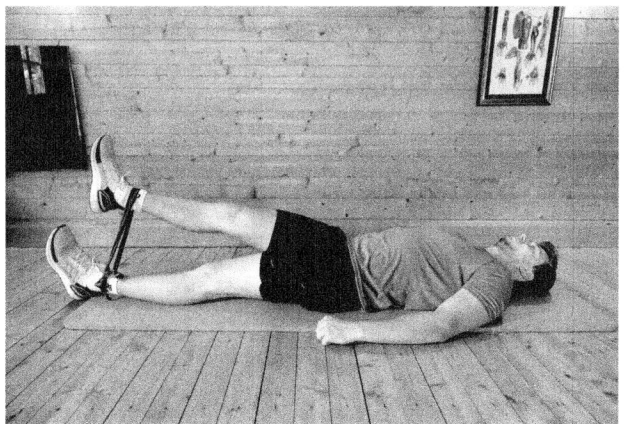

Theraband progession for single leg raises

Standing Hip Extension

This is what is known as an isolation exercise, where just one muscle group is being worked on its own. The gluteus maximus is the muscle which is being worked here.

1. Standing upright, with a stable surface in front of you for support (this can be a table, chair, wall, kitchen work surfaces etc. Make sure you're not stooping when holding onto your surface of choice).
2. To perform the movement, squeeze your bottom muscle and take your hip directly out behind you.
3. Hold the contraction for just 1 second and then return to the starting position.
4. Aim for 3 sets of 10 repetitions with a break in between each set.

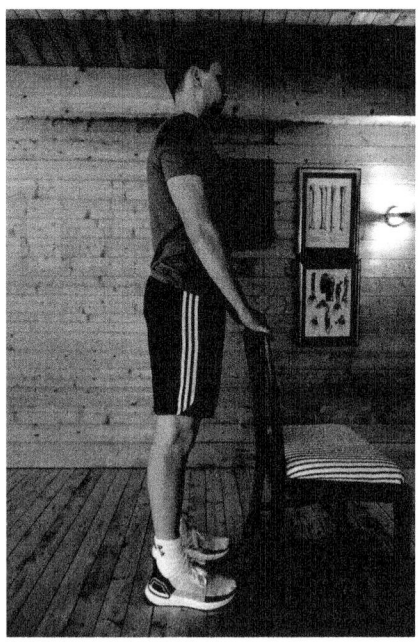

Standing Hip Extension starting position. You can use a chair, wall, table or any other support in front of you.

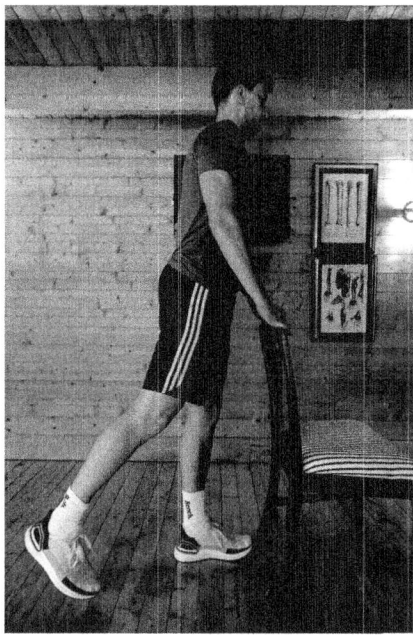

Standing Hip Extension finishing position. Remember not to overarch your back when performing this exercise.

Resistance Band Progression: Loop the band around your ankles and perform the exercise.

Ankle Weight Progression: Yes

Pointers: The main mistake people tend to make with this exercise is over-arching the back which in turn reduces the amount that the glute muscle actually has to work. Keep the back nice and straight when performing the exercise.

Standing Hip Abduction

This exercise is also an isolation exercise but this time just works the gluteus medius muscle which takes the leg out to the side.

1. Standing upright, with a stable surface in front of you for support (This can be a table, chair, wall, kitchen work surfaces etc. Make sure you're not stooping when holding onto your surface of choice).
2. To perform the movement, squeeze your bottom muscle and take your leg out to the side.
3. Hold the contraction for 1 second and then return to the starting position.
4. Aim for 3 sets of 10 repetitions with a break in between each set.

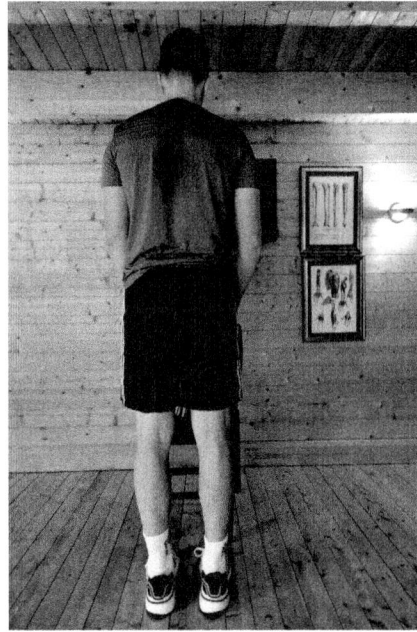

Standing Hip Abduction starting position. This is the same position as the hip extension exercise

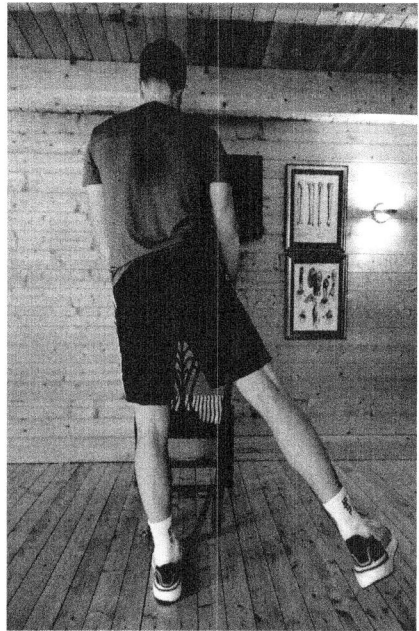

Standing Hip Abduction finishing position. Only take your leg out as far as is comfortable.

Resistance Band Progression: Again loop the band around your ankles and perform the exercise.

Ankle Weight progression: Yes

Pointers: People will often be holding onto a surface which is too low for them causing them to bend over when doing the exercise. This not only puts more pressure on your back but reduces the amount of contraction you get through your glute muscle. Remember to stand up tall when doing this exercise.

Step Ups

This is a great exercise for strengthening your quadriceps, glutes and hamstring muscles all together at once and challenging them on one leg. Developing strong legs when they're working by themselves (i.e. single leg) is important in working towards pain free walking as when you're walking, 50% of the time your leg is on its own. You can use a step on a set of stairs, or a gym fitness step/box.

1. Stand facing a step. Make sure to have a rail or bannister nearby if you feel unsteady on your feet.
2. Step up onto the step with your right foot and to complete the step up there's more technique than you would think.
3. Push through the heel of your right foot and squeeze your right bottom muscle, drive up onto the step while contracting your bottom.
4. Bring the left foot to join your right foot on the step.
5. Return to the starting position by taking your right foot down first.
6. Repeat the exercise by leading with your right foot 10 times (10 reps) and then repeat the exercise leading with your left leg for 10 reps.
7. Aim for 3 sets of 10 reps on both sides with a break in between.

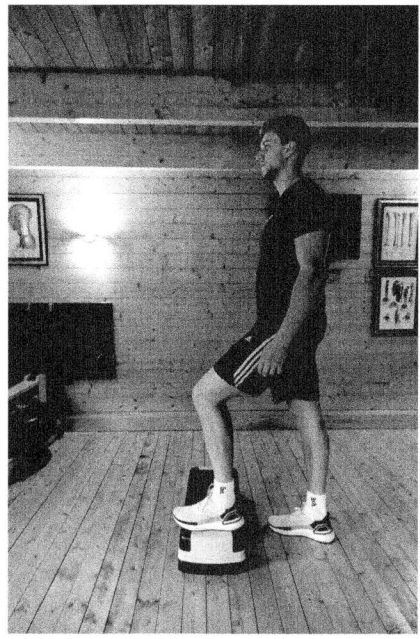

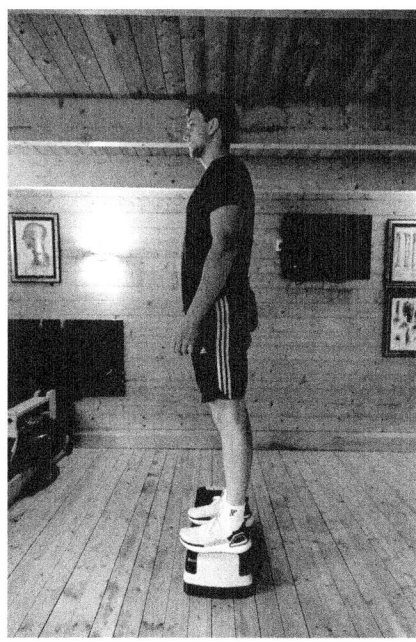

Ankle Weight Progression: Yes

Pointers: I know this might feel a bit silly, just stepping up and down from a step, however if you really focus on contracting the glute muscle when doing it, it is a great exercise to work the muscles of the legs.

Advanced At-Home Leg Exercises

If you find the previous exercises too easy, the following lot are a bit more challenging, and still possible to do at home.

Single Leg Bridge

This is a progression of the *Bridge* exercise we went over in the easy level exercises. It challenges the same muscles but makes it more difficult as there is only a single base of support.

1. Start by lying on your back with one leg bent to 90 degrees and the other straight out in front of you.
2. To perform the movement, engage your core muscles and squeeze your bottom muscles and raise your pelvis off the floor. So your body is angled diagonally. You should feel this in your hamstrings and gluteal muscles.
3. Try to make sure the pelvis is level and is not slanting to one side.
4. Hold for up to 5 seconds (this is a challenging exercise so don't worry if you don't make it to the 5 seconds.)
5. Then slowly return to the starting position.
6. Aim for 10 repetitions of 3 sets on both legs with a break in between.

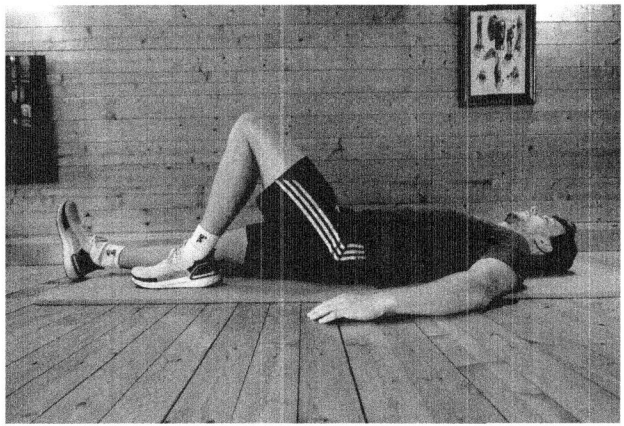

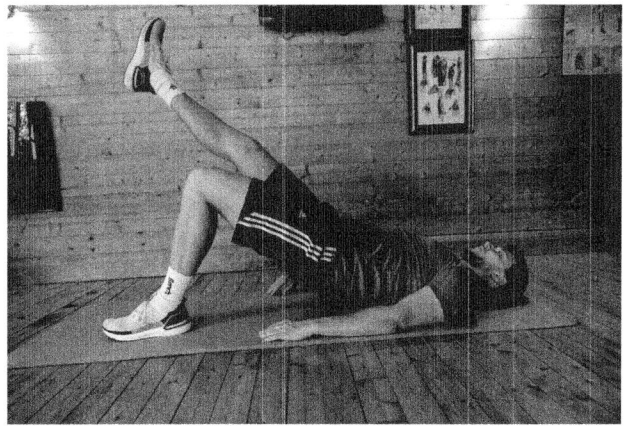

Pointers: Keep your thighs parallel with one another and don't let them drop to one side. Yes it's easier to let one side drop, but for maximum benefit try your best to keep them level.

Squats

Squats are such an important foundational exercise, that if learned how to perform correctly, will help out in so many functional activities. Luckily you have already learned how to do squats in Chapter 3 when learning how to hip hinge! Let's go over the technique again.

1. Stand with legs feet shoulder width apart and feet facing forward.
2. Cross your arms across your chest or have your fists clenched out in front of you.
3. Perform the movement by pushing your hips backwards first and then slowly lowering your bottom down.
4. To return to the starting position, squeeze your bottom muscles and drive up leading with your hips.
5. Aim for 3 sets of 10 repetitions.

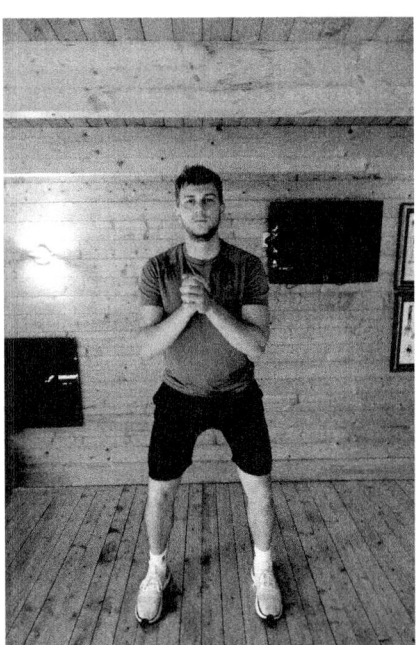

| Squat starting position

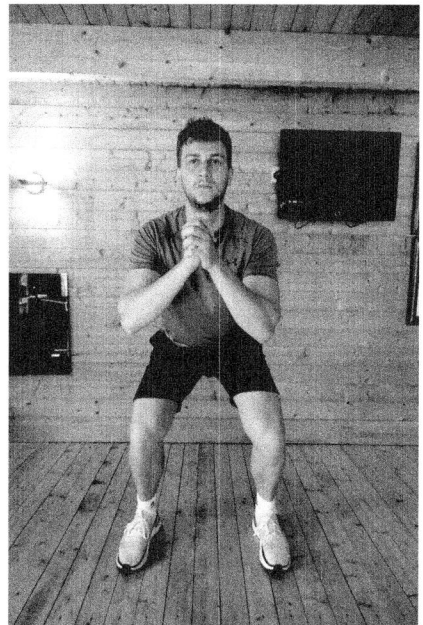

Squat finishing position

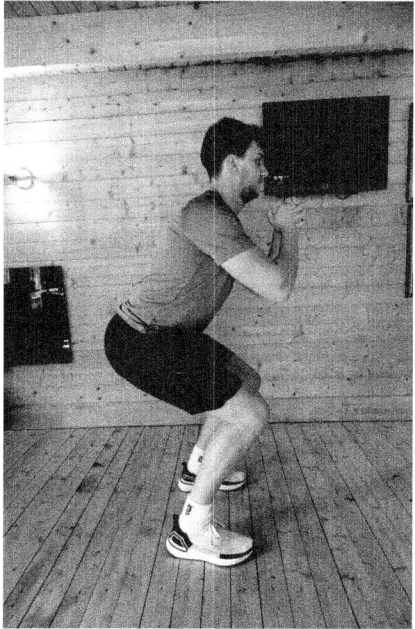

Squat finishing position side view

Resistance band progression: Loop the band around your knees to provide the same effect as with the sit to stand exercises of the band engaging the gluteal muscles more.

Weighted progression: This is particularly useful for those who tend to lean forward when they squat or for those finding the standard squat too easy and need it to be progressed. The exercise is called a goblet squat and is exactly the same but holding a weight with both hands close to your body.

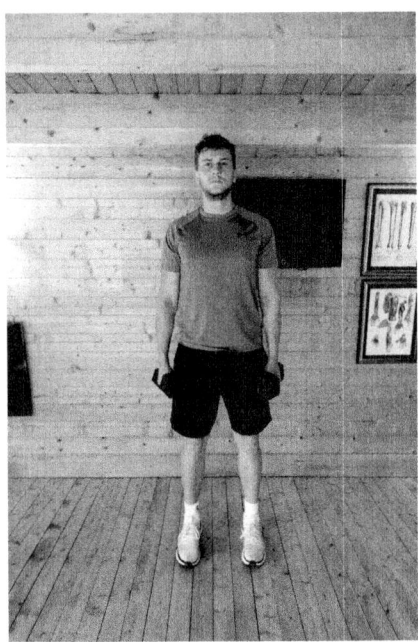

Squat weighted progression with dumbbells – starting progression

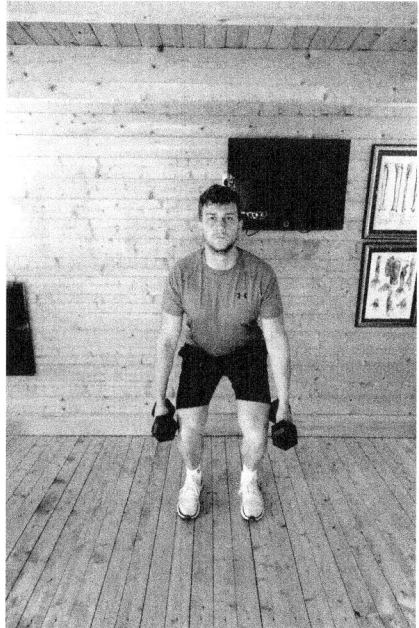

Squat weighted progression with dumbbells – finishing position

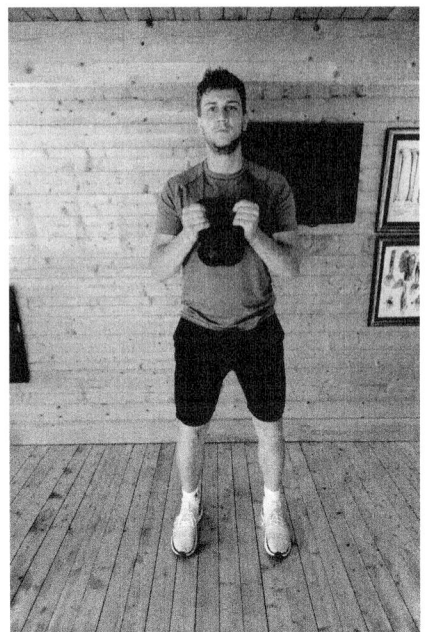

Kettle bell progression

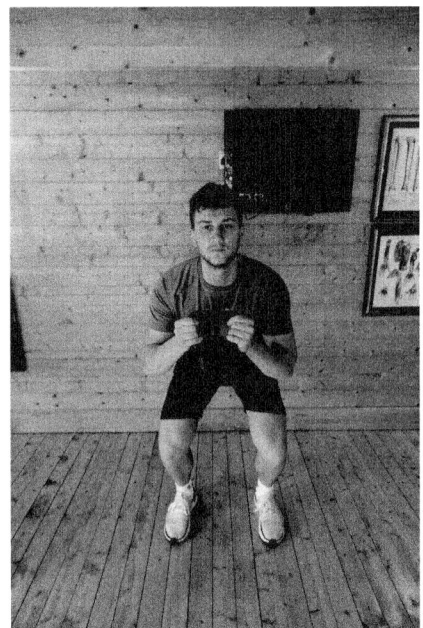

Pointers: There are quite a few pointers to be aware of when it comes to the squat.

- Ensure that the knees track over the toes.
- It's ok for your toes to point outwards slightly, 5-10 degrees of external rotation
- If you notice you are leaning forward when doing a squat it might be caused by your calves/ankles being tight. Try stretching out your calf muscles and ankle mobility for 2-3 weeks by doing the exercises below.

Crab Walk With Resistance Band

As the name would suggest you're going to look like a crab walking when performing this exercise. It's a brilliant exercise for your gluteus medius muscle and also your core gets a good workout as well. You can do this exercise without the band but in truth you won't feel the muscle working nearly as much.

1. Place the band around your knees and stand with feet shoulder width apart and your knees slightly bent. You need a clear space of around 20ft to do this exercise.
2. Engage your core muscles by drawing your tummy towards your spine.
3. Side step to the right 10 steps with your leading leg taking the first step then your trailing leg following behind.
4. You should feel your leading leg glute muscle contract when stepping.
5. After you've completed 10 steps one way, then simply start stepping the other way 10 steps (1 set).

6. Aim to complete 3 sets with a break in between each set.

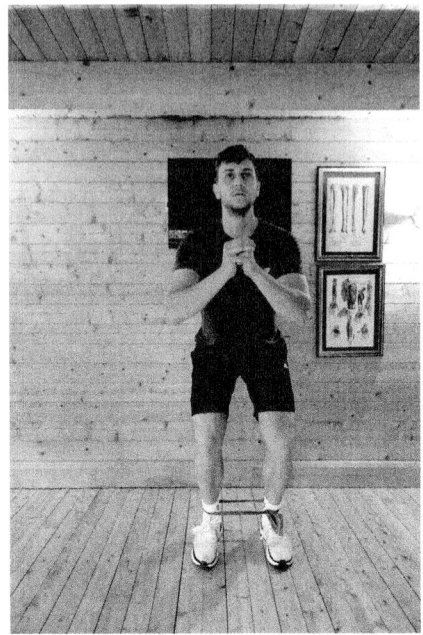

Crab walk starting position – shoulder width apart, with the band pulled taught

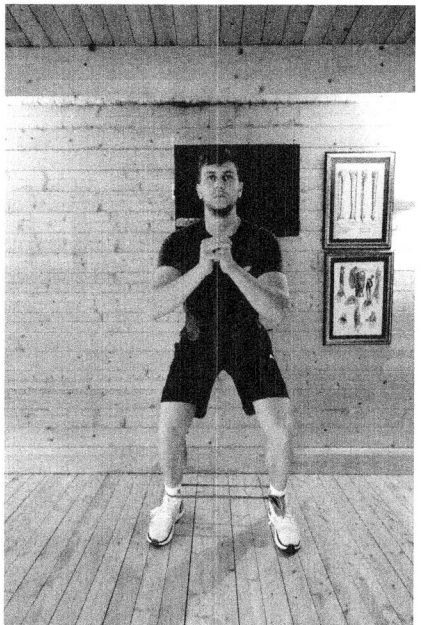

Step out to one side and keep your gluten and core engaged

4-Point Kneeling Hip Extension

Last but certainly not least with the strengthening exercises is the 4 point kneeling hip extension which targets the gluteus maximus muscle. It involves kneeling so if you have dodgy knees then best to stick to the standing hip extension we discussed previously.

1. Start by getting into a 4 point kneeling position with your hands flat on the floor and theraband around your knees.
2. Straighten the knee to be worked out behind you.
3. To perform the exercise, take the foot of the straight leg up off the floor to the horizontal, hold for 2

seconds then slowly lower back down again to the starting position.

4. Repeat on the other side.
5. Aim for 3 sets of 10 repetitions on both sides.

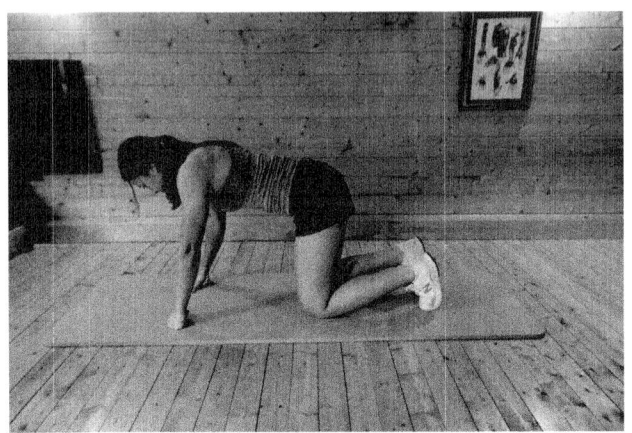

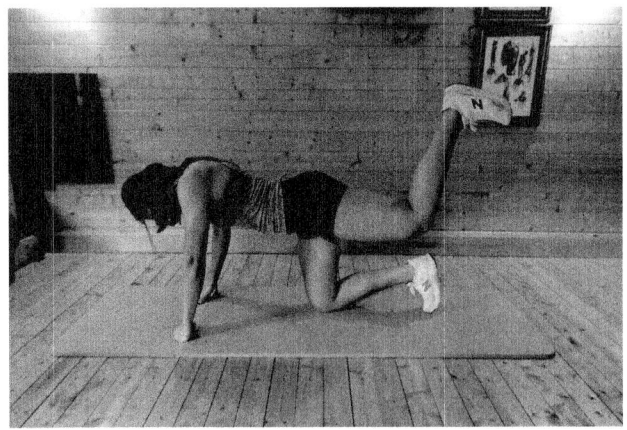

The Gym Exercise Program

The exercises covered here are all straightforward and are resistance machines at the gym. They will work the same main leg muscles that both the 'Easy' and 'Advanced' exercise programs covered. If your gym does not have a particular resistance machine then not to worry, all gyms will have most of the machines discussed here. The instructions will be clearly written on the machines at the gym and if you're struggling with setting it up there will always be gym instructors on site to help you with this, therefore the instructions will be brief.

The Leg Press Machine

There are two types of leg press machines and it's really important you choose the one pictured here. There is another type of leg press where you are closer to the floor and the foot plate that you push rests above you–don't choose this one as it can create much more pressure on your back. In the pictured leg press, you are pushing *yourself* away while in the other type (not pictured), you are pushing *the platform* away. The leg press is a great exercise for strengthening the quadriceps, hamstrings and gluteal muscles.

1. Place both feet on the plate, hip width apart and with your knees bent to roughly 90 degrees. If this is too sore on your back, adjust the seat and move it backwards.
2. Push through your heels and push yourself away from the stationary plate.
3. Perform 3 sets of 12 repetitions. *The weight will have to be adjusted until you find the weight which you can perform 12 reps and 3 sets. Start off with a

low weight and slowly increase. Over-time the goal is to slowly increase the weight but keeping the same reps and sets (12 and 3). If you manage to do this, then that's proof you are getting stronger.

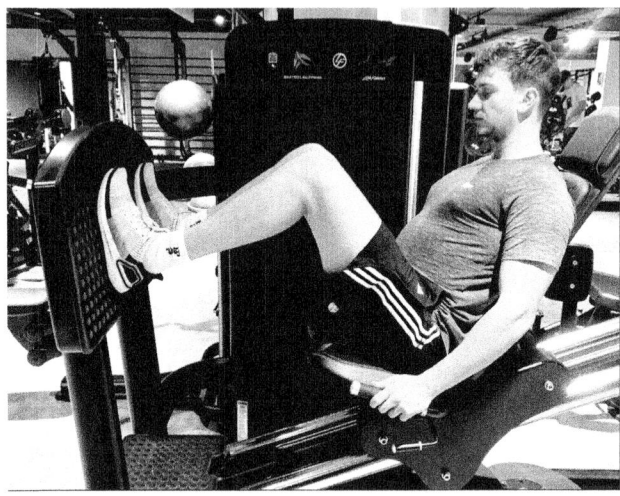

| Leg press machine – Correct starting position

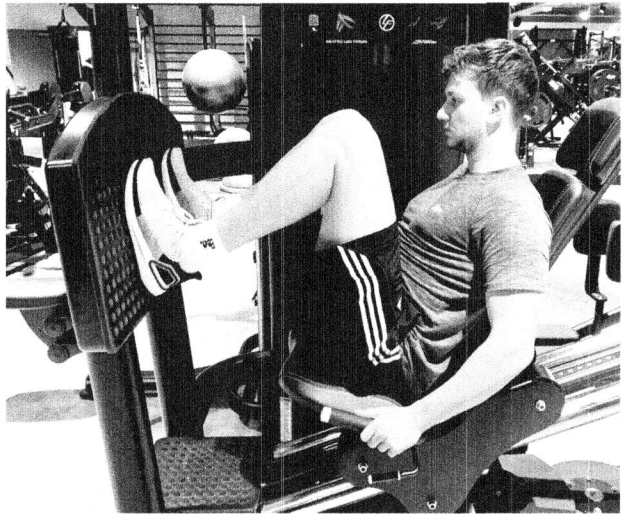

Incorrect starting position – Starting too low is not ideal, as the lower region of the back is curved in this position. This can put increased pressure on the discs when first pushing up, similar to bending and lifting activities.

Knee Extension Machine

This machine isolates the quadriceps muscles (front of thigh muscle) and is fairly easy to use.

1. Sit on the machine with the front of your shins behind the pads.
2. Adjust the seat so the back of your knee creases fit comfortably into the chair.
3. Push the bar away from yourself, you'll feel your quadriceps muscles contracting when performing the exercise.
4. Hold for 2 seconds at the top then slowly lower again.
5. Aim for 3 sets of 12 repetitions.

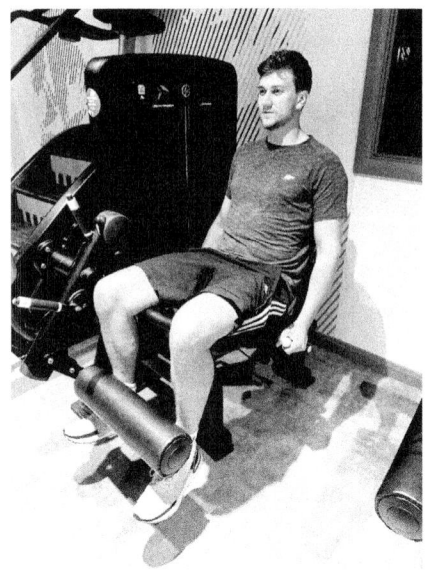

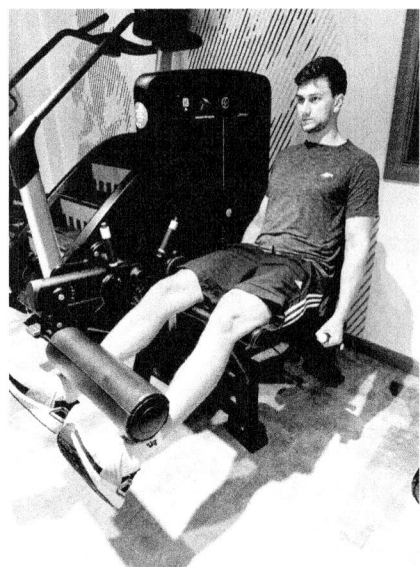

Hamstring Curl Machine

This obviously works the hamstring muscles at the back of

the thigh. The machine is sometimes the same as the knee extension machine and you have to adjust the shin pad and you will still be sitting forwards. *If your machine is that one, then the instructions here don't apply to you. Ask your gym instructor how to change the machine to work the hamstrings and they will be able to show you.

1. Lie on your front with the pad on top of the back of your achilles.
2. To perform, curl the pad up towards your bottom, you will be able to feel your hamstring muscles contract right away.
3. Hold for 1 second at the top then slowly return back to the starting position.
4. Aim for 3 sets of 12 repetitions.

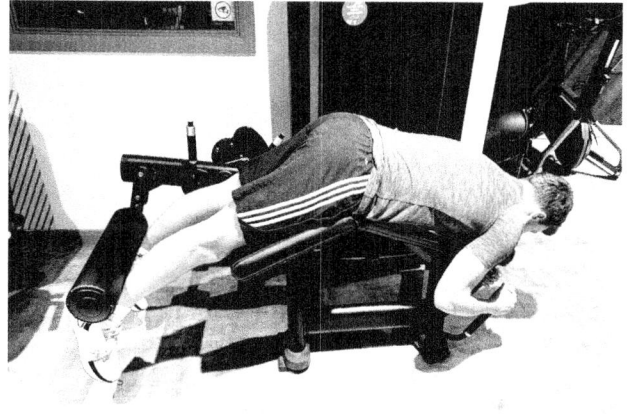

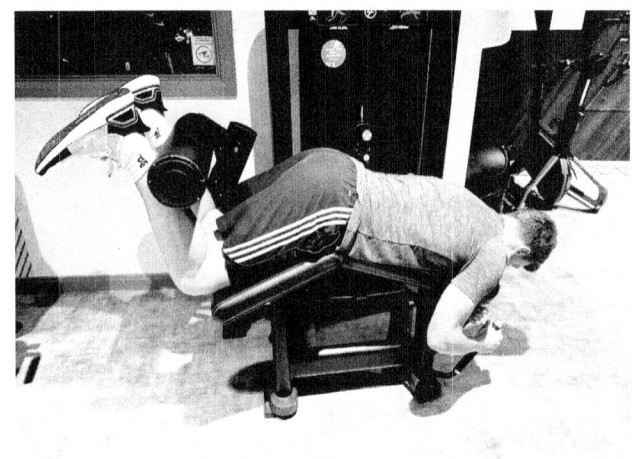

Hip Abductor/Adductor Machine

This machine will nearly always come with both the abductor and adductor in one—you simply need to adjust the pads so they are on different sides of your knees to work the different muscles. To work the inside (*ad*ductor) muscles then the pads need to be on the inside of your knees. To work the outside (*ab*ductor/glute) muscles the pads need to be on the outside of your knees.

1. Sit in the chair and get into the starting position with the pads either on the inside or outside of your knees.
2. To perform the exercise, simply bring the pads together or take them apart from each other.
3. Hold for 1 second and then return back to the starting position.
4. Aim for 3 sets of 12 repetitions.

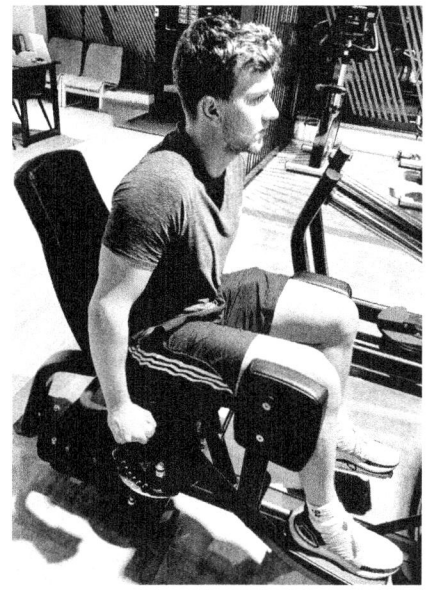

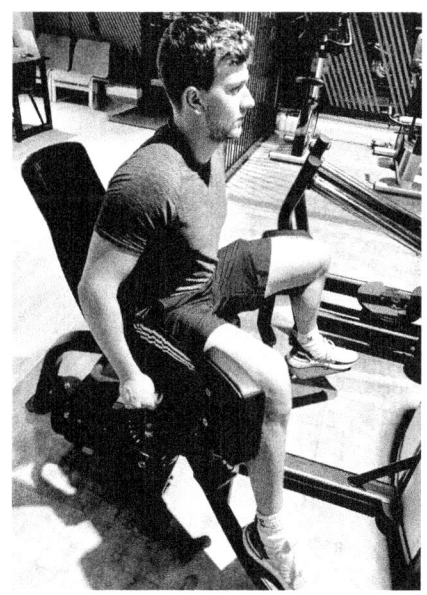

Squats

If you're doing the gym exercise program, you can also incorporate the squats detailed in the previous section, using weights in gym. You can use dumbbells, holding them in each hand, or a single dumbbell or kettlebell holding it with both hands in front of you.

Strengthening Back Muscles

Improving the strength of your back muscles is beneficial in combination with the thoracic stretching exercises previously discussed. Here are two great back strengthening exercises to help correct the posture

Seated Shoulder Horizontal Abduction

This might sound like a very technical name, but it's actually fairly easy to perform.

1. In a seated position, have your arms straight out to the side as shown (please see the supplementary videos).
2. To perform the exercise, bring your shoulder blades together and arms backwards at the same time.
3. Hold this contraction for 10 seconds, then relax (1 rep).
4. Repeat 3 sets of 5 repetitions.

High Arm Row with Resistance Band

For this exercise you will need a long, non-looped band.

1. Loop the band around a stable anchor at shoulder

height. You can either be sitting or standing for this exercise.

2. Bring your elbows up to shoulder height and have your arms straight out in front of you holding onto the band with both hands.

3. To perform the exercise, bring your elbows backwards, squeezing your shoulder blades together. You should feel the muscles in between shoulder blades working.

4. Hold for 1 second and then return back to the starting position.

5. Aim for 3 sets of 12 repetitions with a 45 second break in between each set.

6

Step 6: Cardiovascular Exercises

GETTING STRONGER and getting more flexible seems like a logical step in treating back pain. However, improving your cardiovascular fitness or as I like to put it, getting fitter, seems to be largely viewed as less important. Even among physiotherapists and other healthcare professionals, this part of treating back pain is often overlooked. Once you understand why I preach that it's just as important as stretching and strengthening, I hope you'll make it an integral part of your program. Cardiovascular exercise is any form of physical activity that raises your heart rate above its normal resting rhythm.

3 Key Benefits of Cardiovascular Exercise

1. Cardio mobilizes joints, muscles, ligaments and tendons. If you've picked up anything from this book you will understand the importance of movement for your back. The back doesn't like being in fixed positions for any period of time (apart from sleeping,

which we can't really avoid). Performing cardiovascular exercise is a fantastic way to allow your body (or part of your body) to continuously move, reducing the chance for parts to stiffen and lock up. You only need to perform 10-30 minutes of cardio per day to reap its benefits.

2. It improves your fitness and can help to reduce your weight (in addition to a healthy diet). Increasing your cardiovascular fitness if you're overweight could be the greatest gift you give to your back in losing excess weight, thus relieving pressure from the spine.

3. Lastly, it improves blood flow and nutrients to your spine. Injured tissues, wherever they may be in your body, heal quicker when they have a rich blood supply and regular source of nutrients, and your back is no different. Studies have shown that regular cardiovascular fitness greatly improves both of these factors in your spinal tissues, thus improving the speed of healing.

I can feel the thoughts coming up that might be running through your head–"but I can't run these days!" or, "I used to love swimming but I had to give that up because of my back pain..." I'm here to tell you that there *will* be a cardiovascular exercise out there that you can do that will provide the 3 key benefits we just went through. If possible, the key is to find an exercise which you find enjoyable and manageable, this way you're much more likely to stick to it in the medium to long term.

Some of you won't be able to do all of these cardiovascular exercises, but attempt a few of them, choose your favorite, and then do your best to stick with the ones that you can manage. The main thing is to be consistent with it.

• • •

Stationary Bicycle

- If you're a member of a gym or happen to have one at home, this is a great way to get your legs working and to raise your heart rate at the same time.
- Aim for cycling up to 30 minutes, 2-4 times per week. If that sounds like it might be too long, start with 5 minutes and aim to increase by 5 minutes every week. Progress is progress, no matter how slow.
- Don't have your seat too low, this will round your back too much. The seat should be high enough to allow your thighs to be positioned at a slight angle downwards.
- As you become more confident try and increase the resistance of the bike, again slowly, week by week. This will serve to increase the strength of your leg muscles.
- This form of cardio is particularly good for stenosis sufferers because you are in the flexion position with your back.

Walking

- If you find walking does not make your back painful and actually feels good for it, then walk more!
- Aim for between 15-20 minutes, ideally 2-3 times every day. It is much better for your back to go for 3, 20 minute walks as opposed to 1 hour long walk.
- Remember to swing those arms, shorter and quicker steps if you can.
- If you're walking over rougher terrain e.g. trail walking, and this is causing your back pain to worsen. This is due to the unevenness of the path you're

walking on, not that walking itself is bad for you. If this is the case, stick to solid ground when going out for your walks.

Running

- If you're able to, running is a really great option. When you run, you achieve much greater rotation and general movement through your lumbar spine.
- This may be impossible for some of you but for those whose back pain is not as severe, give it a go and see if it helps.
- As with all the cardiovascular exercises, but especially with running, start slow and gradually increase in terms of both distance and speed.

Swimming

- Both breaststroke and front crawl are good options when it comes to swimming.
- If you can tolerate it, it really is one of the better exercises you can do for your back, as it hits the three important points–it improves your core strength and general whole body strength, your flexibility, and your cardiovascular health.
- It can be a very tiring exercise, so even just starting off with a couple of lengths and slowly increasing the number of lengths can be a great help to your back.
- Those with spondylolisthesis and stenosis will most likely find breast stroke painful for the back due to the extended position the spine goes into.

Foot Pedals

- You can purchase foot pedals online and these are great if you find getting onto a normal stationary bike is too difficult, or you don't have access to one.
- Sitting in a comfortable chair at home, position the foot pedals roughly 1 foot away from you so that you can place both feet inside the pedals. Start pedaling, and aim for 1 minute on and 1 minute off for a total cycling time of 10 minutes. It will take you 20 minutes to complete with the breaks. If that feels too easy, you can reduce the breaks to 30 seconds and double the pedal time to 2 minutes.
- Some foot pedals will have resistance options, and others might not, but the pedaling action itself will provide some benefit in getting your legs moving and raising your heart rate.

Cross Trainer

- If you've ever been to a gym before you will have seen one of these. My patients often ask me if they're safe to use when you have back pain. The short answer is, yes.
- The forwards and backwards motion you get with them provides some great mobility to the lumbar spine without the impact you get when on a treadmill or running. So if you have sore or painful knees, this might be a preferred option.
- There are different resistances you can choose which can make it harder. With an increased resistance this will work your gluteal muscles more, making it a great option for exercise.

Zumba

- The world's most famous dance classes certainly count as good cardiovascular exercise if they can be tolerated. It essentially involves choreographed dance to latin and other international music.
- I must confess I have never attended a Zumba class but when my patients (mainly ladies) ask if it's ok to keep up with the Zumba classes I always advised as long as your back doesn't complain when you're doing it, then keep going!
- Additionally, Zumba is a great way to stretch the fascia throughout your entire body, because you're constantly moving multi-directionally.

Those are the many different ways that you can incorporate cardio into your routine for your back pain management. Don't be afraid to try each of them and choose the one or couple that you enjoy and find manageable, as this will help you remain consistent.

7

Step 7: Consider Other Causes

WHILE I TRULY BELIEVE THAT most cases of back pain can be resolved using the methods in this book, there are a handful of other things that should be considered in addition to working on your stretching and strengthening exercises, and this is the 7th step. This step involves observing emotions, stress, diet, and weight, and it's important to note how these can play a role in the pain we experience.

Emotions and Physical Pain

When we feel pain, it's generally assumed that there is something physically wrong with our body. In the case of back pain, we tend to believe it's usually something along the lines of a pulled muscle, a disc bulge, or some other spinal condition. While this may be the case in most instances, there is also the possibility that the physical pain we are feeling might be attributed to our psychological well-being.

To be clear, in no way is the pain *imaginary* or "all in your head." The pain is very real. However, in some cases, the trigger for this pain might have emotional roots that have led to physical conditions, making the body more inclined to feel pain. As humans, we experience an array of emotions every day, often more negative than positive–stress, anxiety, and sadness can all trigger a physiological domino effect eventually leading to pain and these emotions can play a bigger role than you would think.

When we experience stress, cortisol and adrenaline are released. Our minds and bodies are undeniably connected, and mental thoughts can trigger involuntary physiological responses such as tightening of your muscles, an increased heart rate or breathing rate, or elevated blood pressure. Think about a time when you were told a bit of really concerning news–do you remember how your *body* felt in response to this? Sometimes even just *imagining* a stressful occurrence can lead to these physiological responses.

So when one is experiencing constant stress, or anxiety, these physiological responses will constantly be following suit and creating tension and pain in the muscles in our back. This can often lead to spasms, and the feeling that the muscles in the back are bound and tight. When our muscles become tight, blood flow can become restricted, causing a lack of oxygen in the cells throughout your body. All of these things can then fall into a cycle of pain and stress feeding off of each other. When someone becomes stressed, this can lead to pain. The pain can then lead to inability to perform certain tasks. In turn, the patient will start to feel frustrated and even more stressed that they are unable to move regularly. Less regular movements lead to muscle weakening and inflexibility. This muscle weakening and even less mobility will cause even more stress, and thus, the cycle continues.

Our emotions can also affect other facets of our health. If you've gone through a period in your life where you were emotionally distressed, which I'm sure we all have at one point, you'll likely remember that our responses to that time were not the best. When we enter these periods in our life we often don't sleep very well, our appetites worsen as we eat larger amounts of junk foods, we become easily irritated, and we exercise less. All of these adverse responses caused by our emotions can only make our back pain worse, or at the very least, will delay recovery.

On top of this, the medical community often turns to prescription painkillers or surgery, which raises anxieties and stress, yet again. So you can see how emotions and pain can play into each other. I bet by now you're wondering how to address this issue if your pain *is* potentially caused by emotional stress. Here's what you can do.

1. Be aware. Oftentimes, alleviating an issue can come as a result of knowing the cause of that issue. Once you are aware that it may be past emotional trauma or current stressors that are contributing to your back pain, you can address it more easily and with more conviction, knowing that the real pain you feel is not just "in your head."

2. When we're feeling stressed, or emotionally, drained, one of the best things we can do for ourselves is to let it out. A healthy way of doing this is through journaling. Whether it be pen to paper, or on your laptop, getting the words out in front of you to appreciate what you are feeling, can help relieve stress or whatever emotions you are feeling. Bottling up your emotions can be detrimental for your overall well-being, including both your mental health, and the physical consequences that may come with it. Sometimes simply writing your thoughts and feelings down can help to relieve the pressure you feel from it. However, if journaling isn't enough, you always have

the option of seeking out professional help in the form of a therapist. It's important to see these emotions through and process them, and if a therapist is needed for that, then try a few sessions out and see if you notice any differences in your pain levels. Additionally, exercise, or take up yoga or meditation. These things all can help to reduce the stress in your life, and in turn, pain.

3. Where possible, detox your life of negativity or stress. I know this is easier said than done—wouldn't we all just rid our lives of the things causing us emotional distress if we could? Hear me out though. In some cases, doing what's best for you can reduce a lot of stress. For example, don't take on extra tasks at work or in your personal life if you don't want to, or just can't. It is ok to say no to the things you don't want, or that don't help you. Spreading yourself too thin can cause you to feel worn out, and make you feel less joy when doing the things you *actually* want to do. On top of this, try to keep a clean home. Cluttered and uncomfortable living spaces can cause stress, especially when you get home from stress elsewhere like work. Lastly, and this one can sometimes be a tough one, avoid people who are negative in your life. If they are constantly complaining when they are around you and can never find it in them to at least try and be positive, they are not someone you need in your life. All in all, really try to analyze where the stressors are in your life, and eliminate them where possible. It will make a bigger difference than you think.

Your Diet and Pain

Now that we've talked about how emotions can affect our physical pain, let's go over how nutrition and our diets can factor in. Food is our fuel, and in our best case scenario, we should be fueling our bodies with the best nutrients to help it perform optimally. I've never really liked the analogy of "food is fuel" in the sense that we are like cars, and food is like our gasoline, because it is just not that simple. But, while our bodies are not mechanical machines, they are complex, organic systems that are always changing, and we should treat them as such. We often either feed our bodies too much, or too little, or we eat things that clog our arteries.

While healthy and unhealthy foods exist, we are not talking about food here in the same sense. This is theoretically correct, however, for the purpose of back pain, I am not just speaking about eating healthy as a means for losing weight–although this is another factor which can relieve some of the pressure your back is feeling. There are foods out there that can actually make your pain worse because they increase your body's sensitivity to pain. Some diets, on the other hand, can actually help lessen the pain you feel. Pain is merely a physiological response to external or internal stimuli, and this can be affected by both chemical and physical changes. So depending on the foods you consume, you may feel a noticeable change in its function, and your pain levels.

First and foremost, I want to explain a bit about inflammation in the body. Inflammation has gradually become a more and more common underlying factor in a wide array of ailments, even those that are deadly. In a nutshell, inflammation is an internal form of swelling in the body that is a response to injury, both mild and severe. It can be as minor as a red nose when we have a cold, or as severe as the swelling that comes with a broken bone. However, this inflammation can also occur internally in our organs and different types of tissues. Even our hearts can experience inflammation, and in many cases when someone has a heart attack, inflamamtion will have played a part.

When it comes to our backs, inflammation can affect us in a similar way where it slowly deteriorates our muscles until they can't handle it anymore. Eventually, it gets to a point where the inflammation is just causing the pain, as the pain is our body's way of telling us there is something wrong.

The inflammation itself can play many different roles in back pain. It can show up when we have back injuries like straining a muscle, or herniating a disc, and even when the pain is nerve-related. This increased inflammation can slow the healing process when our circulatory system is overworked. But what do nutrition and diet have to do with this?

Our diets play a role in inflammation because, as mentioned earlier, certain foods can increase inflammation while others can actually improve it. With our current diets, we consume more simple carbs, refined sugars, dairy, and fatty foods than that of our ancestors, and this type of diet encourages inflammation. Instead of filling our bodies with high-nutrient, antioxidant packed foods, we feed ourselves large amounts of sugars and artificial colors and flavors. This just causes more inflammation as our body attempts to balance nutrition and hormone levels.

Additionally, there is an evident correlation between back pain, and unhealthy diets that lead to weight gain, and thus increased pressure on our backs. Excess weight is most generally classified using the body mass index, or BMI. Within the BMI, weight can be classified as underweight, normal/healthy weight, overweight, or obese, and this is calculated through a simple division of the square of height in meters into weight in kilograms. This number does not always tell the whole story, considering some people can be considered overweight even though they are very low in body fat, and just have a lot of muscle mass.

However, as a general rule of thumb, those who fall into the obese category are more likely to display this correlation of back pain and excess weight.

This extra weight creates pressure on the spine and the muscles in the back by having to compensate for the extra weight causing our body's center of gravity to move forward. Additionally, obesity in particular, might indirectly cause someone to get less of the healthy exercise they need, not only to lose weight, but to support a healthy back. Not only does excess fat cause muscle imbalances, but it can also cause even more inflammation. So in order to combat both the weight and the inflammation, your best bet is to stick to an anti-inflammatory diet.

Anti-inflammatory diets consist of fish, nuts, olive oils, lean meats, and avoid high-sugar, refined foods and seed oils (such as sunflower or other nut oils). These types of diets improve your bodies inflammatory response, and help you lower your body fat. But it must be noted that simply eating these foods will not help you lose weight, if you are not also reducing your total caloric intake. You must be consuming less calories than you are burning in order to lose weight, regardless of the type of food you eat. However, if you consume these healthier foods, you will not only have a better chance at losing weight, but it will also help your internal inflammation. Both of these things will in turn help improve your back pain.

Another important thing to note in terms of diet, which is often overlooked, is water intake. Hydration is obviously vital to our survival, and contributes to the body in numerous ways. In between each vertebra of our spine, there are little discs that are composed of mostly water. These discs help to reduce the friction and pressure on our spines. When our body is dehydrated, the discs in our spine become deflated, and are unable to absorb as much shock as it's meant to. This can cause the body to experience pain and swelling in the spine. It's important to stay hydrated, in order to keep our discs hydrated, giving our verte-brae the buffer they need throughout the day. Lastly, when our bodies don't receive enough water, our muscles can "shrivel" which causes our joints to take more of the pressure and friction on themselves, thus causing pain. Drinking enough water is possibly the most simple solution out there, but it may help you more than you'd think, and it's one thing that can't hurt to try!

Putting It All Together

You've made it to the end! I hope you have found it an enjoyable read, but more importantly a *helpful* read with practical tips that you can implement to improve your back pain. Back pain is often treated in a much more complicated manner than I feel it needs to be, and with this book I hope I've somewhat simplified the process for you. Having said that, if you are at all concerned with your symptoms, please go seek medical attention to have a proper physical examination performed and a diagnosis obtained. As I have said, the 7 step action plan is the exact process I take all my patients through when treating them for their back conditions. I prefer to keep things simple when treating back pain and uniformly go through the 7 holistic steps I have created. I make sure my patients have ticked all of the boxes! If they have, I know I can feel confident that they are setting themselves up for their best possible outcome. In some cases, you may need to get your severe pain under control before thinking about rehabilitating. However, when you have achieved pain control or when you feel as though you are in a place to engage in rehabilitation, then this book will be a great starting point.

As I mentioned earlier, I have created supplementary videos to go alongside the book.

To access them, head over to:
  basics.chrisrawsonphysio.com

If you have found this book and the programs to be helpful, I would greatly appreciate if you could head over to Amazon to leave a review!

To leave a review, click right here.
  Alternatively, just head over to the book's page on Amazon and scroll down to the link where it says "Write a Customer Review."

Your support is greatly appreciated!

The exercise program you saw at the start of the book is below. The important points are as follows, as the table is on the next page:

- Fascia stretches are to be done 3x daily.
- Stretching (5 exercises, 3 days per week). Choose between either a lumbar flexion stretch or a lumbar extension stretch alongside the lumbar rotation, hamstring, gluteal/piriformis and hip flexor stretches.
- Core exercises: Choose either the Easy or Advanced program, twice per week.
- Leg strengthening: 3x per week. To choose either home easy, home advanced or gym program.
- Postural exercises: 2x per week, if you feel this is required. You can do some back strengthening exercises, work on your standing posture, hip hinging

(recommended for everyone!), or thoracic spine stretches.

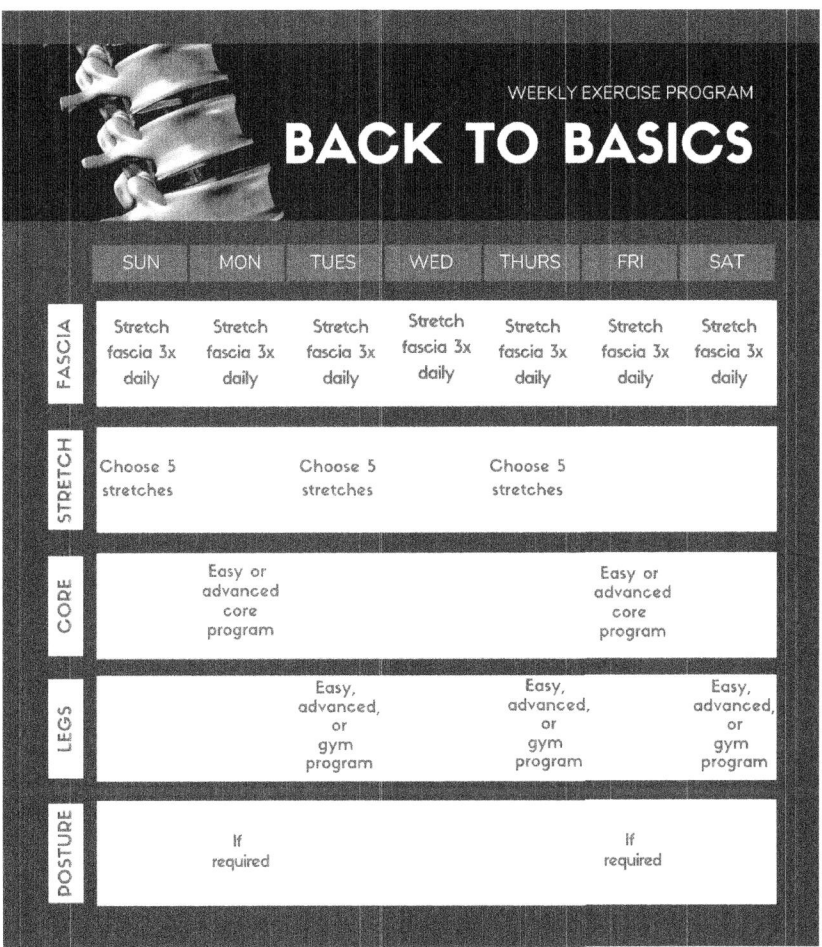

	SUN	MON	TUES	WED	THURS	FRI	SAT
FASCIA	Stretch fascia 3x daily	Stretch fascia 3x daily	Stretch fascia 3x daily	Stretch fascia 3x daily	Stretch fascia 3x daily	Stretch fascia 3x daily	Stretch fascia 3x daily
STRETCH	Choose 5 stretches		Choose 5 stretches		Choose 5 stretches		
CORE		Easy or advanced core program				Easy or advanced core program	
LEGS			Easy, advanced, or gym program		Easy, advanced, or gym program		Easy, advanced, or gym program
POSTURE		If required				If required	

WEEKLY EXERCISE PROGRAM **BACK TO BASICS**

If any of the exercises you are doing are painful or making your back pain worse then please stop them. Where possible try to increase either the resistance or difficulty of the core, leg strengthening or back strengthening exercises this will improve your strength. Over time, with consistency, and applying what you've learned through this book, I hope that your pain will improve and you will be better equipped for managing it. Good luck, and I will see you in the videos!

Printed in Great Britain
by Amazon